The Best Way to Stay Healthy

Stay As Far Away From Doctors As You Can!

Volume I:
The Mediterranean Hunter-Gatherer Diet

Never Experience Hunger
Slow Aging as You Lose Inches
Eliminate Heartburn and Diabetes

George H. Steele Jr, MD

Never visit a doctor
until you are one hundred years old

An old Russian proverb

First Edition June 2003
Greenway Press Incorporated
Merion, PA

NOTICE

This book is a source of information for improving your health but, for more serious conditions, it cannot serve as replacement for the services of a licensed health care professional.

If you suspect you have a medical problem, you should not only seek competent medical advice, you should educate yourself about the nature of your illness and treatments. Any application of the material set forth in the following pages is at the reader's discretion and sole responsibility.

A Note from the Author: December 3, 2003

   Thank you for purchasing this book. My hope is you will find some helpful tools for living life. This is Volume One. This section is dedicated to *Staying Healthy* and how to accomplish this by focusing on what we put in our bodies. Volume Two (to be released soon) will be directed at healing; healing our body, mind and spirit. My suggestion is to try to implement many or most of the changes presented here in Volume One. If you continue to not feel terrific, then it may be time to look at Volume Two: *Healing*. It is important to seek the help of your physician if you are not improving as you may have already developed a significant health problem. But my hope for all of us is that we will continue to be healthy in body, mind and spirit for as long as we desire.

   If you would like to purchase additional copies of *The Best Way to Stay Healthy,* please visit:

http://www.lulu.com/GeorgeSteeleMD

George H. Steele, Jr., M.D.

To Kathy

CONTENTS

VOLUME I: STAYING HEALTHY

VOLUME II: HEALING
(To be released soon)

PREFACE TO VOLUME I

Staying healthy requires us to do each of the following:

First, understand our bodies

Then, understand what causes our aging

We need to change some of the foods we are eating (avoiding the foods of famine) and understand why we must do this to be and stay healthy

We also need to examine our attitudes and learn to accept ourselves as we are so we may live a positive life with power rather than a negative destructive life

And finally, we will explore interventions to alleviate problems we have already developed

1   Understand Your Body

The foundation of our health is our genetic inheritance, but nutrition, toxins, infections, accidents, and finally, our attitude have a significant effect on how our genetic predisposition is manifest. During my nineteen years as an Internal Medicine physician and educator, it has become clear to me that modifying our environment and the foods we eat is the best way to stay healthy.

Your Lifestyle Accounts for 75% of Your Risk of Disease and Death

Environment and nutrition are much more important in determining our health than our genetic inheritance, appearing to account for 75 percent of disease occurrence while genetics accounts for 25 percent.[1] This book will try to optimize the 75 percent of this risk that is modifiable. While we may not be masters of our fate, we can at least give ourselves the best odds and feel great while we are doing it! This is the best way to stay healthy.

2   Understand Your Aging (Chapter 2)

This book approaches aging as postponing the inevitable (and staying healthy in the meantime). The question is asked, what causes us to age? And then again, aging starts in our twenties, followed by more questions and answers (see glossary on page 21):

Why do our joints ache?

Why do we wrinkle?

How does insulin promote disease and early death?

What are superoxide radicals and how do they cause disease?

---

[1] Verkasalo PK, Kaprio J, Koskenvuo M, Pukkala E. Int J Cancer 1999 Dec 10;83(6):743-749 Genetic predisposition, environment and cancer incidence: a nationwide twin study in Finland, 1976-1995.

What is apoptosis?

What is glycation?

We will answer each of these questions, and more, in terms of the inevitability of aging and how to best *stay healthy* in the meantime.

3   Avoid the Food of Famine (Chapters 3 through 6)

As you understand the significant adverse effects caused by consuming sugars, starches and certain fats, your motivation for eating changes. Instead of eating to meet our cravings, we choose foods that make us feel strong, clear-headed and positive. Most people who reach that point will never sink back to eating the foods of famine (better known as junk food or better yet, dog food filler).

The Seven-Day Plan of Nutrition for Women (Men, you will eat 50% more; as if that is fair!) is designed to keep our bodies running smoothly for most of the potential 130 years of life. It is also grain-free and avoids the proteins and sugars from dairy, which can be associated with adverse reactions in many people.

If we truly understand that how we feel today (and the rate of our aging) is directly related to the food we eat – we find it easier to *just say no* to the morning bagel (this book calls it *Bagel Death*). If we also understand that if we feel terrific right now, we are much more likely to feel terrific in five to ten years. If we feel lousy now, imagine how we might feel in five to ten years. Now is the time to feel great. Now is the time to slow aging, so let's do it!

4   The Mediterranean Hunter-Gatherer Diet (Chapters 7 & 8)

This book explains which foods are in, which are out and why. The specifics of the Mediterranean diet are explored, beginning with a Seven-Day Plan of Nutrition for Women. This plan presents a strategy for implementing changes in your eating habits to reduce insulin resistance and thereby reduce your risks for heart disease, diabetes, cancer, depression, and early death (with numerous options-including slow-suicide options for days you get up on the wrong side of the bed). You will find recipes to get you started for breakfast, lunch, dinner, dessert and snacks. There are complete weekly menus and recipes accompanied by nutritional breakdowns (fat, protein, carbohydrates, fiber, omega-3 oils and cholesterol) for each dish, and shopping guides. Men can carry out this same plan by simply eating 50% more of the same foods (this may not seem fair but who said life was meant to be fair?)

5   The Mediterranean Hunter-Gatherer diet versus the Atkins', Ornish and Protein Power (Chapter 9)

The Atkins' diet has been shown to reduce all heart disease risk factors but the saturated fat may promote shrinking of your brain (small vessel disease in the brain). But the ketosis in the very-low-carbohydrate diets (Atkins', Mediterranean Hunter-Gatherer, and Neanderthin) may actually reduce aging. The other low carbohydrate diets (as opposed to very-low-carbohydrate diet) including Protein Power, South Beach, Sugar Busters, The Zone, etc. do not allow ketosis and therefore may not be as helpful in reducing aging.

6   Nutritional Supplements can be Helpful or Harmful (Chapter 10)

A few supplements can actually reduce your risk of diabetes, heart disease, cancer and arthritis (chromium, fish oils, and MSM-methylsulfonylmethane). Others may actually increase diabetes (glucosamine) or high blood pressure (St. John's Wort) or cancer (possibly Saw Palmetto?) or heart disease (taking Vitamin E capsules showed a trend toward worsening heart disease). So I encourage patients to eat a healthy and varied diet with the good oils and lots of nuts, green vegetables, eggs, fish and lean meats and poultry.

7   Ultimate Sports Nutrition (Chapter 11)

Burning fat as fuel allows you to exercise longer and harder while consuming less oxygen (hence less breathing required) and thereby less oxidative stress (aging). Sugar requires more oxygen to burn and may actually harm tissues as you exercise.

8   Asthma And Allergies Can Be Optional (Chapter 12)

This book looks at the causes and treatment of allergies. Milk makes more mucus, so if you are congested avoid milk, cheese, yogurt, ice cream, and pizza. Other foods that can contribute to congestion include the sulfites in wine and vinegar, orange juice and other citrus, chocolate, soy, peanuts, and wheat. All of these foods appear to stimulate the immune system in an adverse way promoting an over-reaction to environmental allergens. Avoiding these foods can greatly reduce symptoms of allergic rhinitis, chronic sinusitis and asthma, and is often much easier than avoiding dust, mold, mildew, animal dander and pollens.

9   Eating Wheat Promotes Certain Illnesses (Chapter 13)

The protein in wheat (gluten) irritates the lining of the intestines in many people and may worsen inflammatory bowel disease (Ulcerative colitis and Crohn's disease), allergies and asthma, as well as Celiac Sprue and Irritable Bowel Syndrome.

10   Alcohol: the Two-Edged Sword (Chapter 14)

A little alcohol is better than none-at-all and a lot better than too much (more than 9 drinks per week for women and 14 drinks per week for men) in reducing heart disease and cardiac death. But the risks of drinking may outweigh the benefits so be careful and drink moderately if at all.

But Does This Actually Work?

In the last two weeks I have had two obese patients return to see me after four months on the Mediterranean Hunter-Gatherer diet. Each had recently developed diabetes with a hemoglobin A1c (test of diabetes control) over 13mg% (a tremendously high level). In four months, the first fellow had lost 50 pounds and five inches while the second lost 60 pounds and six inches (albeit from a 44 to a 38). And both had healed their diabetes (their A1c levels are now normal).

But many patients do not succeed. They seem to be held back by some unknown force (perhaps a negative attitude?). The purpose of the second volume of this book is for people not succeeding in meeting their goals of health and purpose in life. First is *Volume I: Staying Healthy* that contains important nutritional information for all of us. For those of us who continue to struggle despite having studied Volume I, *Volume II: Healing* will provide more tools and suggestions to move us toward greater health.

PREFACE TO VOLUME 2

Staying healthy requires us to do each of the following:

First, understand our bodies

Then, understand what causes our aging

We need to change some of the foods we are eating (avoid the foods of famine) and understand why we must do this to be and stay healthy

We also need to examine our attitudes and learn to accept ourselves as we are so we may live a positive life with power rather than a negative destructive life

And finally, we can incorporate needed interventions to alleviate problems we have already developed

In Volume 1 we explored aging and how a large waist predicts health problems such as diabetes, cancer and heart disease. Then we discussed how in starving yourself (dieting) you lose muscle as well as fat (but you don't want to lose muscle), while if you reduce calories by eliminating sugar and starch you actually gain muscle and lose only fat.

The Mediterranean Hunter-Gatherer diet was presented as one way to become lean and healthy again. This diet is rich in the healthy oils including fish oils, nut oils, olive oil and grapeseed oil as well as others. It also encourages eating whole foods and lots of green leafy vegetables as well as meat, fish and poultry and some nuts and berries.

Whereas Volume 1 focused on creating a healthy body, the essence of Volume 2 is to encourage us to accept ourselves as already healed. In that act can we begin to actually heal our mind, body and spirit. Fear and guilt harm our bodies. The Trappist monks referred to fear and guilt as the 8th and 9th deadly sins, producing separation of each of us from God, our communities, and even ourselves.

1   Examine Your Attitudes (Chapters 15 & 16)

The premise of this book is that most of us fail to stay healthy not because of lack of knowledge but from a negative attitude. It is clear that hostility is highly associated with heart disease[2] as is depression with early death.[3] This book provides tools to help us understand who we are and what we can do to stay healthy.

Attitude is the key. But how do we overcome a negative attitude? Fear can lead to anger; guilt can lead to depression. Only by letting go of our fears and guilt can we begin healing. It is not enough to know what to eat and how to exercise. We must love ourselves enough to put good food into our bodies and lead healthy and active lives.

---

[2] Williams RB. A 69-Year-Old Man with Anger and Angina. JAMA 1999, 282:763-770.
[3] Wulsin LR. Does Depression Kill? Arch Intern Med 2000, 160:1731-2.

2   Incorporate Interventions to Get Rid of Specific Diseases (Chapter 17)

These include the common cold, diabetes, hypertension, high cholesterol, arthritis, congestive heart failure, and depression. This book makes clear how an optimal diet and positive attitude can both supply the basic needs of the body and fortify the body's defenses and mechanisms of healing to stay healthy.

(a)   *Breast, Prostate, Colon, And Lung Cancer*

Insulin and sugar accelerate the growth of prostate cancer (as well as colon, breast and pancreatic cancer). This book explains how one of the most effective treatments for advanced prostate cancer is a low-sugar/low-calorie diet. Changing your lifestyle can reduce breast cancer recurrence by a factor of eight while keeping you healthful and hopeful.

(b)   *Arthritis and other problems when our bodies attack themselves*

Why do our bodies attack and destroy our joints? This does not make sense. Something in our environment turns on our immune systems and then turns our immune systems against our joints. Infections such as Lyme Disease and Parvovirus B-19 do this. But it is also true that certain foods contain proteins (lectins and others) that stimulate the immune system to destroy our joints. Avoiding corn, certain other grains and the nightshade vegetables (eggplant, potatoes, peppers and tomatoes) may help some of us avoid or reduce arthritis.

Are your ankles and feet sore when you first get up in the morning? Do you have to hold the railing to walk down the stairs? There is a supplement called MSM (which is similar to glucosamine but appears to be better at reducing pain) which can alleviate most of these symptoms. Insuring adequate dietary sulfur appears to be key to having healthy connective tissue (shown in studies of supplementation with glucosamine and methylsulfonylmethane -MSM).

(c)   *Chronic Fatigue Syndrome*

Chronic fatigue syndrome is a good example of what can go awry when our mind and body react to our environment in an adverse way. We will look at both conventional as well as integrative medicine treatment and explain the rationale behind each.

(d)   *Iron Storage Disease Can Be Suppressed By Regular Blood Donations*

Iron storage disease (hemachromatosis) is the most commonly inherited disease, which promotes heart failure, diabetes, and liver disease. Most people consume excess iron. However, if you donate blood regularly and have your ferritin checked (a blood test), the manifestations of this disease can usually be avoided.

(e) *Obesity*

Increased waist circumference (over 30 inches in women and 35 inches in men) is associated with increased insulin resistance which can lead to diabetes, heart disease, cancer and depression (and early death in worms and rats). The very-low-carbohydrate diet lowers insulin levels and has been successful in many patients in reducing their waist circumference and its attendant risks.

(f) *Accidents*

Perhaps you have heard it stated that there are no accidents. We become distracted by issues of life and ignore the world (and people) around us. If we focus on the needs of others and ourselves (especially while driving- instead of the cell phone or the radio), we will find we can hear the future in many situations and thereby avoid accidents.

3 Diabetes Can Be Made To Go Away! (Chapter 18)

The goal of this book is not to treat diabetes but to get rid of it (you really don't need it). Many people with Type 2 diabetes can resolve their hyperglycemia (high blood sugar) by eating the Mediterranean Hunter-Gatherer diet; patients with juvenile diabetes (Type 1) can also benefit. The interventions in this book also prevent diabetes from developing in the first place in people at increased risk. This includes those people with a waist circumference greater than 33 inches in men (28 inches in women) measured at the point of your stomach that enters the room first (usually near the belly button).

4 Hypertension and High Cholesterol are often A Lifestyle Issue (Chapter 19)

Hypertension is often a lifestyle issue, not a lack of the right medication. In some people it is stress, or foods containing allergens (particularly wheat and alcoholic beverages), or the lack of appropriate exercise. Meditation, exercise, changing the foods you eat, and forgiveness of yourself and others (letting go of anger and resentment) can have a major impact on your blood pressure.

Elevated LDL cholesterol is most frequently associated with elevated fat stores and elevated insulin levels and greatly reduced by changing these underlying risk factors through changes in eating habits. In the one out of twenty patients with genetically high cholesterol, there are specific recommendations on how to diagnose and treat. If your LDL-cholesterol is very high or if you have diabetes, you will need to limit or avoid egg yolks, shrimp, lobster and fatty meats. For those people with normal cholesterol levels, eggs with runny yolks appear to promote health.

5   Depression Is A Chemical Imbalance (Chapter 20)

Depression is a chemical imbalance that can be improved by antidepressants, chromium picolinate, avoidance of sugar and starch, eating a very-low-carbohydrate (ketogenic) diet, and forgiveness of yourself and others. If you can avoid the antidepressants by doing the other interventions, your sex life will undoubtedly be better.

6   Sex and Spirituality (Chapter 22)

My favorite section is entitled Searching for an Effective Spiritual Placebo (section 6 in Chapter 22), which explores the three kinds of devotion, recognizing our suffering, the three doors of Hell, psychic masochism, and the stages of life. There is a little poetry (by yours truly) and a few stories as well.

7   The Appendices

These provide the specific tools for healing discussed in the chapters listed above. Included are the Emotional Freedom Technique (EFT), Relaxation with mental imagery, Relaxation with the autogenic (affecting your nervous system) technique and a summary of the Enneagram: the nine ways of responding to stress.

What is the Absolute Minimum I Recommend?

Some of you do not want to spend any more time than absolutely necessary to accomplish feeling better and living longer and healthier. The minimum I suggest is as follows. Remember that eating sugar is death!

Eat green leafy vegetables, olive oil, tree nuts (like almonds, walnuts, pecans, Brazil nuts and cashews), fish/eggs/poultry/meat, berries and alcohol (if you drink alcohol) in about that order. If you are not trying to lose weight, you may add some non-citrus low-sugar fruits, oats, black beans, lentils and maybe a little rice (if you are starving but only if you do not have heartburn).

Avoid all wheat products (bread, pasta, pizza, etc.), processed fruit juices, and limit or avoid most sugar and starches (elevated insulin and blood sugar greatly promote heart disease and cancer).

Milk makes more mucus in most of us, so if you or your family have allergies or asthma, avoid the protein (casein) in milk, cheese, yogurt, ice cream, and pizza.

Eat fatty fish (herring, sardines, or salmon) three times per week (better than Coral Calcium!) (Or you may take the mint or lemon flavored Cod liver oil).

Take calcium citrate 500-1,000mg with vitamin D 400-800 units per day. If you take the Cod liver oil, do not take extra vitamin D. Take magnesium citrate 250-500mg (helps bones and the heart) and chromium polynicotinate 200mcg once daily (older rodents given chromium behave like younger rodents. Can you imagine what that might mean?).

Take MSM 3,000-4,000 mg once in the morning if you are not drinking rainwater and eating living things (MSM relieves the aches and pains of getting older, not to mention reducing wrinkles and keeping your hair and nails healthy).

Exercise regularly (Take the stairs, empty the dishwasher, take out the trash, and then take the dog for a walk- a complete physical fitness program).

Have a significant person or pet (a dog is good; a partner is better but unfortunately it appears that taking on a husband may shorten your life but perhaps some would consider it worth the trouble?).

Practice forgiveness, of yourself and others (particularly your spouse).

Avoid too much media exposure (TV, radio, newspapers, magazines, the Internet, and the local gossip); it may distract you from who you are and what you can do with and for the people around you.

Wear a hat in the sun to protect your eyes (reduces cataracts and macular degeneration).

Wear your seatbelt (and turn off the cell-phone and radio so you can listen to the world around you).

Do not try to make others happy, but share your happiness with others (make yourself happy in life today).

These suggestions are designed to keep you healthy. If you are not feeling better after trying these lifestyle modifications, please go back to your doctor, as you may need more evaluation and treatment for problems that have already developed.

Glossary of Important Terms

Apoptosis (A-pop-**toe**-sis): my absolute favorite word, which means our bodies are designed to die at a certain time, i.e. 130 years of age (programmed cell death, or pop goes the cell). Our cells live only so long and then die. This can happen sooner if you develop diabetes or a large waist (more than 35 inches in women, 40 inches in men). You want to delay apoptosis for as long you can. Get your waist smaller and avoid sugar, starch and cigarettes.

Atherosclerosis (Aa-ther-o-skler-**o**-sis): this is hardening of your arteries leading to heart attack and stroke (to be avoided if possible). Keep your waist small (below 35 inches for men and below 30 inches for women) and your LDL cholesterol below 100 mg%.

Autoimmune (auto-im-**you**-n): this is your body attacking itself, which is a bad thing. Try to avoid foods and infections that stimulate our bodies to over-react to normal situations (more about this in the allergy section of the book).

Carbon monoxide: cigarette smoking causes wrinkles due to the carbon monoxide in the cigarette smoke; wrinkles of your face as well as your heart muscle, your kidneys, and your blood vessels (meaning you are aging). Don't smoke, or if you do, smoke Lucky Strike non-filters (lower in carbon monoxide). But you know those must be bad for you!

Celiac disease (See-lee-**ak**): the protein in wheat flour causes the immune system to destroy the lining of the small intestine in approximately 1% of the US population. It increases the risk of small bowel cancer by fifty times, as well as reducing absorption of important nutrients. We do not need to eat wheat flour (unless we are crossing the desert).

Crohn's disease (Krone's): another disease in which the immune system attacks the intestines. No cause is known but many patients improve if they avoid grains, dairy and yeast (see Chapter 13).

Diabetes (Die-a-**bee**-tees): this term means to urinate too much (in this case due to too much sugar in the blood). Most patients with diabetes have type 2 diabetes, due to eating too much sugar and starch causing their waist to grow too much (more than 35 inches in women, more than 40 inches in men are high-risk measurements). Avoid the sugars and starches and lose the waist.

Gene (Jeen): the DNA or chromosomes that carrying the code for who we are going to be. But we can mess this code up by living too wild (smoking, eating excess sugar, etc.).

Glucose (**Glue**-kos): the sugar in your food and in your blood.

Glycation (Gly-**kay**-shun): this is where sugar acts like glue making all of our tissues stiff and old. This is seen in patients with diabetes or people with a large waist and elevated blood sugars. Avoid the starches and slow aging.

Glycemic (Gly-**seem**-ik) Index: a measure of how much a food with raise your blood sugar and insulin level (and thereby increase stiffness, aging and the growth of tumors).

Insulin (**In**-sue-lynn): the hormone that tries to keep our blood sugars in a narrow range (not too little and not too much). But eating excess sugar and starch leads to higher insulin levels which increases weight gain, diabetes, heart disease and cancer.

Ketosis (Key-**toe**-sis): when you are burning fat your body make ketones for fuel. You can measure if you are burning fat by seeing if there are ketones in your urine (using the Ketostix, see Chapter 11). In ketosis you lose only fat and actually gain muscle).

Mitochondria (My-toe-**kon**-dree-a): the part of the cell that creates chemical energy to allow the cell to function and repair itself. If the mitochondria are damaged (by oxidative stress or the burning of too much sugar), then the cell cannot repair itself and will die before it's time.

Oxidation (Ox-i-**day**-shun): excess oxygen being used by the cell, which leads to damage to structures in the cell and eventually can lead to premature cell death.

Dr. Steele is on the faculty of the University of Pennsylvania School of Medicine in the Division of General Internal Medicine. His previous appointments have included faculty positions at Duke University, Brown University, the University of North Carolina, and the Medical College of Pennsylvania (previously the Women's Medical College of Philadelphia). His areas of interest are the impact of nutrition on health and metabolism, as well as the impact of attitude and emotions on health and well being. His next project is finishing Volume II of this set, which will focus on healing of the mind, body and spirit (all of which comes from within, of course).

First, Do No Harm

Hippocrates

1

STAYING HEALTHY

**1   The Best Way To Stay Healthy Is To Stay As Far Away From Doctors
As You Can**

First, Do No Harm

The Hippocratic Oath states this clearly and overtly.
It says nothing about making patients better. Yet we often risk harm to do good.

My interpretation of the Hippocratic oath is as follows:

Impart knowledge
Instill hope

(Then check to be sure that the patient understands because people get confused)
(And before proceeding, don't forget to make sure nothing is already wrong!)

Physicians:
(We can all be physicians and healers)

A healing attitude is the key to success
Eat the *Mediterranean Hunter-Gatherer Diet*
Find some exercise you like and do it
Wear a hat and don't get sunburned!
Wear comfortable shoes
(Eat sardines?)

Physician, heal thyself!

If you feel better when you do this, then suggest others do the same!

Promises I make to myself
I am healing
I put good things into my body
I have money to give away
I have love to give away
I try to be present in every minute of every day

(a)   *The Meaning of Illness*

Our symptoms and diseases are our bodies telling us something is out of whack. Sometimes it is a subtle message, like tightness in our neck and shoulders, or aching in a joint. Other times it is the warning shot across the bow of our ship of life when we develop depression, diabetes, heart disease, or cancer. This warning indicates that a major life change is mandatory. If we listen to our bodies, we will hear what is *off* and be able to address it. Often the problem arises from something we are putting into our body, or from something we are not putting into our body (we are what we eat). At times it may be related to our approach to life.

I believe in healing. I believe if people understand how their lifestyle affects their body and how they feel (now), they will make better choices- especially if they have better choices- nuts, good fruits and vegetables, moderate alcohol consumption, and Starbucks' Decaf.

I also believe in aging. I see it every day in myself, in my family, and in my patients. Occasionally I can even see into the future. This occurs when I see patients who remind me of someone who has not done well. They are choosing a path that is a slippery slope to early death.

Yet it can seem so simple. Your face reflects the health of your whole body. Is your face looking older? Then your body is aging also. If your skin is getting stiff, wrinkled, and non-pliable, then the same process is occurring in your blood vessels, your heart muscles, and your joints. They are getting stiff, wrinkled, and non-pliable.

(b) *What Causes These Wrinkles and Other Abnormalities of Our Skin and Internal Organs?*

- *Insulin resistance*: insulin acts as a growth factor promoting the growth of fat cells, tumor cells,[4] and atherosclerosis[5] (cholesterol plaques in your blood vessels). This growth promotes early death through such diseases as diabetes, heart disease, stroke, and cancers of the prostate, breast, colon, and pancreas.

- *Glycation:* much of the stiffness of our tissues originates from the excess sugar in our system acting as a molecular glue sticking proteins together making them stiff and yellow.[6] The most obvious place to see this is in the wrinkles on our faces. This can also be appreciated in the stiffness of our joints as we age. The same process is occurring in the lenses of our eyes resulting in our arms needing to get longer and our glasses slipping to the end of our noses. What is harder to appreciate is that our blood vessels and our heart are also getting stiff and old.

- *Carbon monoxide (and other toxins) and oxidative stress:* we once thought that the major adverse effect of carbon monoxide was to reduce the ability of the blood to carry oxygen. Recent work at Duke University has revealed that even low levels of carbon monoxide poison the metabolism of the cells of our body and greatly increase oxidative stress by blocking pathways that reduce super-oxide radicals. This promotes aging of our skin (wrinkles), aging of our brain (dementia), and aging of our lungs (emphysema and lung cancer). So stop smoking already!

- *Autoimmune phenomenon:* This is where our bodies are attacking themselves. Our puffy faces, our aching joints, and our irritable intestines often signify more than we give them credit. Inflammation underlies most serious illness, yet we ignore many symptoms that signify that our immune systems are turned on in an unhealthy way.

We are starting a journey to understanding our own aging and how to optimize it. So how do you feel today? Like it or not, this accurately predicts your long-term outcomes. If you're looking and feeling great today, chances are in five years and ten years you will also feel great. But if you are not feeling well today, just imagine how bad you will feel in five years. Now is the time to change course.

---

[4] Hilf R, Livingston JN, Crofton DH. Effects of diabetes and sex steroid hormones on insulin receptor tyrosine kinase activity in R3230AC mammary adenocarcinomas. *Cancer Res* 1988 Jul 1;48(13):3742-50.

[5] O'Keefe JH, Miles JM, Harris WH, Moe RM, McCallister BD. Improving the adversecardiovascular prognosis of Type 2 diabetes. *Mayo Clin Proc* 1999;74:171-180.

[6] Viassara H. Advanced glycosylation in diabetic nephropathy and aging. *Adv Nephrol Necker Hosp* 1996;25:303.

If you go to five doctors, you will get five opinions (and they may all be wrong!). You must find your own solutions that make sense to you. I spend much of my time with sick people trying to figure out what works and what doesn't.

(c)   *A Few Rules That May Help:*

- First do no harm (don't do anything too risky)
- Don't go to a doctor who smokes
- Don't go to a doctor who is overweight
- Don't go to a doctor who is chronically stressed
- Don't go to a doctor who is truly unhappy

A good doctor is better than a bad doctor

and almost as good as no doctor at all

Anonymous

An unhealthy doctor can not be a healer. Physician, heal thyself-first! If they can't even do that, they have no business in the business of the practice of medicine. In 1997, I came to the realization that I had been harming patients telling them to eat the American Heart Association diet!

Dear Father O'Hara:

How do I convince thee that potatoes promote aging and that bread is the staff of death?

We are all physicians; we are all healers. We are all able to find a path to healing, first for ourselves, and then by example we can help those around us. But not until we begin to solve our own problems can we help others. Many of my patients have become healers, some despite having no interest in becoming one. But through their excitement in living and feeling great, others are drawn to them seeking answers for their ills. They share their knowledge; they share their hope.

But some of us have yet to awaken the healer within us. Yet that healer is in all of us. We must help each other to find the hope, the knowledge and the healing.

The following paragraphs will illustrate my evolution as a physician in the exam room:

- From conventional to integrative
- From practice guidelines to food and exercise suggestions
- From back operations and knee surgery to Tai Chi and massage

(d)   *Avoid Becoming A Patient on the Conveyor Belt of Disease Management*

Here are some common examples:

- Diabetes Type 2
- Asthma
- Crohn's Disease
- Celiac Disease

Disease management protocols are a consensus approach to a problem, which is usually the most conservative (but not necessarily the most effective) approach.

- ***Diabetes Type 2***: The medical community and the disease management protocols are just beginning to approach Diabetes Type 2 as a problem of insulin resistance and the dysfunctional modern diet. Most of the emphasis in the past has been on using oral medications and insulin to overcome the effects of the high starch diet the patients were consuming. In the attempt to lower blood sugars, we were causing further weight gain, even more insulin resistance, and actually a higher risk of cardiovascular death. Again it was felt that a diet like the Hunter-Gatherer Diet was unworkable for most patients. So we took the easy way out and gave these patients more and more medications. Some patients were given hundreds of units of insulin per day, which did little to overcome their insulin resistance and instead prompted even greater weight gain and complications. An intelligent Diabetes doctor from UNC taught me that it makes no sense to give patients with Diabetes more than 60 units of insulin per day. Instead he would bring the family in with the patient and hang crepe as in a funeral. This doctor would tell the family that the patient had a very serious (almost malignant) disease and needed to radically change the patient's approach to life, both in what the patient ate and how much they exercised. Sure, this didn't always work, but at least he wasn't just enabling the patient and family to continue in the path toward early death. If they chose not to, so be it, and vice versa. Part of the reason I have spent so much time trying to create a workable diet is I believe what we eat is the foundation of how we feel and how we age.

- ***Asthma***: Today a patient (who also happens to be a pediatrician) called me for an exacerbation of asthma. I asked him if he knew that milk makes more mucus. He told me that he was quite aware of the fact, and avoided all dairy products if he was having an exacerbation. He had trained in Seattle with Gail Shapiro, MD who has done extensive work on the effect of food sensitivities on allergies and asthma. I complained to him that many do not seem to know about the effect of diet on allergies. I have never seen a monograph on asthma that mentioned anything about diet and asthma (they are always pushing medications-why would they include information that might make the medications appear less useful?).

- *Crohn's disease*: This is a disease of inflammation of the whole intestinal tract (one of the inflammatory bowel diseases). I attended the Internal Medicine Update at Harvard Medical in the fall of 2001. There was a talk on Inflammatory Bowel Disease(IBD), during which the professor spent much time on the use of medications in the disease. Fortunately, in the handout, there were abstracts of articles about the treatment of Inflammatory Bowel Disease. Two of these articles discussed the use of diet in the treatment of Crohn's disease. One discussed the use of an elemental diet in patients with steroid refractive disease (not responding to even the most aggressive conventional therapy).[7] Ninety percent of the patients had remission of symptoms by removing grains and dairy from their diet. My two patients with Crohn's have had their disease go into complete remission using *The Mediterranean Hunter-Gatherer Diet*. Now the conventional medical approach considers using bone marrow transplantation to treat Crohn's. These physicians are the same individuals who suggest that a strict diet without grains or dairy is unworkable. But what they may not be completely honest about is that a diet without grains or dairy probably never killed anyone, but autologous bone marrow transplantation has a small but finite risk of death.

- *Celiac Disease* (Gluten-Sensitive Enteropathy): one out of every 100-200 people has Celiac Sprue. This is a disease in which the proteins in wheat cause inflammation in the small intestine leading to poor absorption of nutrients, stomach pain, diarrhea, and other problems including lymphoma and arthritis. Most physicians do not give Celiac disease much thought because it is felt that the treatment (a very strict grain-free/gluten-free diet) is very difficult and usually unworkable. Yet many people suffer with intractable intestinal problems even into their 70's because we are not looking for this disease. Even in my practice of 3,000 patients I have only diagnosed 5 patients with Celiac Sprue. Which means I need to find the 10 to 20 others with Celiac disease. Although if my patients follow the Mediterranean Hunter-Gatherer Diet, they will not have any problems as this is gluten-free (except the occasional wheat starch used in processed or prepared foods). The conventional recommendation for patients with Celiac disease tends to be a very high sugar diet. I believe people can do better than eating marshmallows and drinking Coke (both gluten-free and fat-free but very unhealthy). That is why I suggest the Mediterranean Hunter-Gatherer Diet.

---

[7] Hunter JO. Nutritional factors in inflammatory bowel disease. *Eur J Gastroenterol Hepatol* 1998 Mar;10(3):235-7.

So what happened to the healing arts? Can you avoid this conveyor belt of disease management? Instead of managing your disease, how about listening to your body (for once!) and making your disease go away. Is your doctor trained to help you do this?

No.

(e) *The Response of Conventional Medicine*

If you have a problem, we have the following possible responses:

- We order a blood test or two
- We prescribe a pill or three
- We issue a referral to a specialist who will look at you as a shoulder or a stomach or a heart or a colon or a nut case
- We will order a diagnostic procedure on you to find out what's wrong
- We will do surgery to get you better (because we can fix your shoulder or back or knee or nose)

It is time to have an open mind; it is time to seek solutions outside of the conventional answers. We need to rediscover how to deal with higher levels of uncertainty in our practice of medicine. We used to be able to do this. We used to do much less testing and treated patients first with a therapeutic trial. An example of this includes trying physical therapy for knee problems instead of MRI scan and knee surgery. Another is doing a stress test and cardiac rehabilitation following a heart attack instead of cardiac catheterization and angioplasty (they put a tube into your heart and use a balloon to dilate your blood vessels) because using this balloon dilation has not been shown to prolong life.

It turns out that most of the lumbar laminectomies (back operations) done over the last 30 years did not need to be done (close to 90% according to estimates by the Rand Group) because surgery did not appear to improve outcomes when assessed at 7 years. The same appears to be true of many of the knee surgeries. Most patients improve and can return to normal function with aggressive rehabilitation instead of surgery. The patients who definitely need surgery are those with locking, giving way, and/or significant recurrent swelling of their knees.

(f)   *Thinking Outside the Box*

Is your face looking older? Of course it is, but why? The answer is simple:

- Glycation: sugar molecules binding to proteins in your skin (and blood vessels, heart muscles, etc.) cause the proteins to cross link making the tissues stiff and yellow.

- Oxidative damage: The appearance of aging in your face mirrors the aging of your whole body. Let us take smokers for an example. Carbon monoxide from cigarette smoke (and other sources) greatly promotes oxidative stress not only causing wrinkles in your face but the aging of your body. The carbon monoxide blocks a critical pathway the body uses to degrade superoxide radicals, the chemical complexes that destroy bacteria, viruses, and normal cells that get in the way. If these complexes build up in your system, they cause damage and cell death.

- Auto-Immune Phenomenon: Our immune system attacking our tissues because of toxins we ingest or because our immune systems become out of balance due to certain proteins in our diet (sulfites in wine, peanuts, or milk protein) or infections we contract (such as Lyme disease, mycoplasma and Parvovirus B-19).

- A negative attitude and belief in aging rather than healing.

(g)   *A New Look At Old Problems*

But do not reach for the Retin A yet- that is cheating, and only masks the underlying process and gives you the false impression you are beating the system. But imagine trying to get your face healthier by living and eating right. You might not consider that worthwhile unless the changes actually allow you to feel better now, and in five, ten, twenty years.

Successful aging is predicted by the following, according to the Harvard Study on Aging:[8]
- Highly satisfying life partnership with spouse or significant other
- Highly satisfying relationships with your children and/or friends
- Highly satisfying income-producing work
- A sense of humor when things are not quite working out the way you wanted

---

[8] Vaillant GE. *Aging Well*. (Boston: Little Brown, 2002).

2   Negative Attitudes Lead to Negative Effects on the Body

A rabbit heart disease study comes to mind. Dr. Cornhill studied a group of rabbits that were bred to develop atherosclerotic heart disease (hardening of the arteries).[9] Two-thirds of the rabbits at autopsy had severe heart disease but a third did not. It was finally determined that the third of rabbits that did not develop heart disease were the rabbits that had been in the cages in the middle row (not the top or bottom rows). One of the technicians caring for the rabbits routinely took the middle row rabbits out of their cages to play with them. The others were left in their cages. The results were duplicated in a subsequent study. When I told this to a friend of mine, he turned away shaking his head muttering *Then I'm dead.* Evidently his wife does not take my friend out of his cage often enough to caress and play with him.

(a)   *Men and Stress*

Men are a lot like rabbits; we need to be taken out of our cages sometimes and cuddled. But the same is true of the female of the species. So whatever it takes to get your relationship with your life-partner on a better footing, do it. It will be worth it. If you need help relating to and appreciating your spouse, see Appendix Five in Volume 2 for the nine ways we respond to stress. If you can come to appreciate that when your spouse is stressed out s/he becomes angry, belligerent, hostile and controlling, you will stop taking it personally every time they explode. You will instead put your arm around them and ask them *what is wrong, dear?* Yeah, right. But it works.

3   Positive Attitudes Lead to Positive Effects on the Body

(a)   *Family Life Predicts Longevity*

A good relationship with our children and/or friends requires us to let them be themselves. Play to their strengths and support them in their struggles. Sometimes we need to let go of our aspirations for them and help them reach for their *own* goals successfully. A patient suggested the advice for stressed parents of college age students and older: *Hold them close with open arms.*

---

[9] Nerem RM, Alevesque MJ, Cornhill JF. Social environment as a factor in diet-induced atherosclerosis. *Science* 208(4451):1475-6, 1980 Jun 27.

(b) *Work Is Good For You*

Meaningful paying work can occur anywhere doing almost anything in a community that you value and trust. Be it art, medicine, business, music, childrearing, teaching, counseling, or spiritual leadership, ask for what you need and stick to your list. Do not sell yourself short. Open your eyes to the needs of others and society and fill those needs (after establishing adequate financial backing, of course).

(c) *Laughter: The Best Medicine*

Humor is the key to survival. Make fun of how bad things seem to be. It can take the edge off. Work together with others to enhance the situation. But always try to sustain your sense of humor. The most successful old person I've met is a 96 year old man who has had both recurrent colon cancer and bladder cancer, not to mention breaking his back several times (vertebral compression fractures) from falling. He still rolls his own cigarettes using pipe tobacco and drinks George Dickel whiskey as well as the occasional Dos Equis. He has never lost his sense of humor despite all of the physical insults (among others) he has suffered. He has also continued to work as a children's book illustrator and was remarried 13 years ago to a women in her late 40's. A month before they were married, she caught him in bed with another woman (a woman from the hair salon at that). His fiancée said *How could you do this to me?* He explained that it was nothing against her but that when an unmarried man his age (then 83 years old) gets an offer like that he just has to take it. She accepted that, took him as he was, and their marriage together has been wonderful. They have remained devoted to each other. Both are remarkable people.

Excess Insulin and Sugar Promote Aging and Early Death

If you don't super-size your fries and soda,
How are you ever going to get to be 300 pounds?

A Fast Food Worker

2

AGING: POSTPONING THE INEVITABLE

1 Are You Feeling Great?

So, are you feeling great? If not, why not? If you feel tired, why are you so tired? If you feel tired today, imagine how you might feel in five to ten years? It won't be pretty. But how can you make such a tremendous change in your life as growing younger when you feel less than great? Have you seen people jogging and wondered how they had the energy? Have you tried innumerable times to start exercising (punishing?) but after several days stopped because *What was the point; I still don't feel well?*

(a) *How do we get past the fatigue and malaise?*

Listen to your feelings, your body. *If you are not feeling great, there is something wrong.* Our bodies are designed to perform at a high level almost indefinitely (approximately 130 years is the best estimate), and some individuals almost accomplish this. What is wrong with the rest of us? Are we not as good people? Is it some psychological problem we are unable to circumvent? Is struggling through life our destiny?

Actually, we all create our own destinies through our thoughts and actions. We have a choice, but we must start listening to our bodies and trusting ourselves and how we are feeling. Much of what we have been led to believe is not true. *What is good to eat? What is not good to eat?* There is little evidence at this time to support the low fat diet, which has made many people not feel well for so long. It is time we started thinking for ourselves and trusting our feelings and our bodies.

(b) *What could be causing this fatigue we experience?*

Most of us push our bodies hard, working too much, staying up too late, eating just to keep going. If we are tired, we often do not rest, but instead reach for something to keep us going. Coffee, Coke, chocolate, alcohol, whatever. But this fatigue does not arise from working too hard. It arises from the chronic over-release of adrenaline that accompanies our lives. What causes these high adrenaline levels? It is not what you think. Psychological stresses account for some of this, but many people also suffer from insulin resistance with high insulin levels and/or chronic allergic conditions. At least some of this arises from our diets. In this book we will explore what causes higher insulin levels and what it does to our bodies. We will also look at chronic allergies and their impact on health and aging.

2   The Problems of Aging

Aging continues on a daily basis, but we can slow the inevitable. In the table below are listed some of the major problems of aging. By understanding what is causing these problems, we can begin to address the various underlying etiologies before they steal away our health and longevity.

Look carefully at the following table to determine what problems of aging are most problematic for you. Then study their cause. We will look at the top nine ways to reduce aging. When you know which are the most important you will know where you need to focus and which ones you can play with a little.

TABLE 2-1: PROBLEMS OF AGING

Problems of Aging	Underlying Causes
Weak muscles (reduced muscle mass)	Inadequate or unbalanced nutrition (particularly protein deficiency and chromium deficiency) Lack of resistive exercise
Brittle bones (osteoporosis)	Inadequate nutrition (magnesium and calcium) Lack of resistive and weight bearing exercise Smoking / excess alcohol use Vitamin K deficiency / Vitamin D deficiency
Stiff blood vessels (atherosclerosis leading to heart attacks and strokes)	Vascular inflammation leading to atherosclerosis (diabetes, IGT, homocysteine, infections, oxidized LDL cholesterol) Excess iron; Vitamin K deficiency
Cancer of breast, prostate, colon, pancreas	Growth factors for tumors (insulin and insulin-like growth factors <IGF> from diabetes and impaired glucose tolerance <IGT>), Nitrites (colon)
Cancer of lung, colon, cervix, throat, esophagus, and bladder	Tissue inflammation leading to precancerous changes and cancer (smoking, nitrites, distilled liquors consumed undiluted, ?smoked fish)
Slowed nerve function (peripheral neuropathy leading to poor balance and numb feet)	Diabetes and impaired glucose tolerance (IGT) Vitamin B-12 deficiency Low thyroid function Toxins (excess alcohol)

Stiff heart (cardiomyopathy leading to congestive heart failure, atrial fibrillation and other arrhythmias)	Diabetes and impaired glucose tolerance (causing excess glycation- glucose acting as molecular glue) Hypertension (from stress, sleep apnea, allergies) Excess alcohol; magnesium deficiency Excess iron
Liver disease	Excess alcohol Excess iron Chronic viral hepatitis
Reduced kidney function (renal insufficiency)	Hypertension Diabetes and impaired glucose tolerance
Joint pains (arthritis)	Autoimmune inflammation arising from infections such as Lyme disease and Mycoplasma (walking pneumonia); reaction to inflammatory bowel disease or psoriasis; gout; Nightshade vegetables? Diabetes and IGT (frozen shoulder); excess iron
Enlarged prostate (BPH)	The $64,000 question (Is insulin a growth factor? It appears to be at least for prostate cancer)
Reduced vision (macular degeneration and cataracts)	Impaired absorption and vitamin deficiency (Vitamin B-12, vitamin D, lutein, Vitamin K, chromium) Diabetes and impaired glucose tolerance
Loss of memory (Alzheimer's and other neuro-degenerative diseases)	Mitochondrial gene deletions due to oxidative stress Toxic exposures (smoking and excess alcohol) Infections (Mad cow disease, Cruetzfeld-Jacob) Vitamin K deficiency Diabetes and impaired glucose tolerance

As You Go Through This List, A Few Things Jump Out

- Diabetes and Impaired Glucose Tolerance (IGT or pre-diabetes) appear frequently.
- Nutrition seems to have more importance than we give it credit.
- Arthritis (which may be preventable) cripples our ability to act young and active to maintain muscle and bone health
- Inflammation is bad, be it in blood vessels, joints, intestines, liver or lungs.

- Cigarette smoking is bad (causing wrinkles inside and out)
- Alcohol is a two-edged sword
- Donating blood is healthy (eliminates excess iron and checks for chronic liver disease)

If we could avoid whatever it is that causes our joints to become inflamed, we should be able to avoid or at least postpone arthritis. Could it possibly be certain foods (corn consumption is associated with arthritis in dogs) or infections (Lyme disease and Parvovirus B-19 for example) or nutritional deficiency (the supplementation of sulfur in glucosamine and MSM improves arthritis)?

Is your face wrinkling? Sure it is, but don't use Retin-A (the acne medicine that improves wrinkles) or get Botox injections. Your face is a good indicator of internal aging through the processes of glycation (sugar acting as molecular glue) and oxidative stress, not to mention apoptosis (programmed cell death when the cell just runs out of time and energy). But to fully appreciate the wrinkles in your face you must understand what is causing them. Only then will you be able to begin to heal them and slow further wrinkling.

A few key concepts to understand as we undertake growing younger and reduce wrinkling in a healthy way for the whole body.

(a)   *To Be Stiff Is To Be Old*

Glycation: sugar acting as molecular glue, making all of our tissues stiff and yellow. This stiffening occurs in the skin (which we can see) as well as our heart, muscles, blood vessels, joints, and intestines. One of the major differences between the young and old is the pliability of our tissues. To be stiff is to be old. Much of this stiffness is due to glycation. To avoid excess sugar, Diabetes, and Impaired Glucose Tolerance (IGT), we can markedly reduce the accumulation of this glue that slows us down.

(b)   *Light Cigarettes cause more Damage than the old short Lucky Strike?*

Oxidative stress from super-oxide radicals (also known as reactive oxygen species): Our bodies use these super-energy oxygen molecules to destroy bacteria, viruses, and damaged tissues. They are therefore useful substances when in the correct setting. The problem arises when they accumulate inappropriately in the cell and begin to damage the structure of the cell itself.

Super-oxide radicals are a byproduct of the metabolism of glucose. When we burn sugar as fuel we create more oxidative stress. The body has many mechanisms for absorbing this energy and turning it back into safer, lower-energy molecules, but this requires the presence of significant amounts of anti-oxidant molecules to recycle the energy. Two problems can occur: we deplete our anti-oxidant molecules or we consume substances that block our ability to recycle this energy safely. One of the main substances that block this recycling is carbon monoxide in cigarette smoke and automobile exhaust.

Light (and ultralight) cigarettes produce much less tar (tar causes chronic lung disease) and nicotine (associated with the addiction). The flip side is they produce much more carbon monoxide per nicotine dose than the old heavy cigarettes. Since people smoke for the nicotine, they are receiving much higher doses of carbon monoxide to maintain their therapeutic nicotine level. Physicians used to think that low levels of carbon monoxide were not bad because there was still plenty of oxygen being carried to important organs by the blood. Recently, however, researchers at Duke University discovered that even low levels of carbon monoxide block the recycling of super-oxide radicals and thereby cause significant oxidative damage in all cells.

Cahill has shown that when the body burns fat as fuel (the ketogenic diet; both the Atkins' and the Mediterranean Hunter-Gatherer diets are ketogenic), the main byproducts are carbon dioxide and water.[10] This is like burning natural gas (a much cleaner fuel burning to carbon dioxide and water) instead of gasoline (which has numerous toxic byproducts). Therefore it appears that not only is the body more efficient burning fat as fuel, this may be the anti-aging approach because of the reduced oxidative stress.

As these super-oxide radicals accumulate, damage begins to occur. The worst of this is deletion of important genes (DNA) in our mitochondria (the parts inside our cells that make the energy for the cell to work and repair itself; pronounced my-toe-**kon**-dree-a).

(c)   *Eve and the Loss of Eden: Mitochondrial Gene Deletion*

We call her Eve.[11] She was born in central Africa 73,000 years ago. It is believed we are all related to Eve through our mitochondria, the powerhouse of our cells. We receive all of our mitochondria from our mothers in the cytoplasm of her egg. The father's sperm only provides half of our body's genes but no mitochondria. We know we are related to Eve because Eve's mitochondria have more similarities to the mitochondria of people around the world than any other prehistoric person found. Mitochondria have their own DNA (they were probably once free living parasites that infected the cells of our ancestors). If damaged they do not produce enough chemical energy making the cell less able to repair itself.

(1)   Why are Mitochondrial so Important?

Our cells are constantly being damaged by our environment and by what we eat and don't eat. We are constantly producing cancer cells, and constantly killing cancer cells. We are constantly repairing and replacing most of our bodies. ***We need tremendous amounts of chemical energy to do this***. We count on our mitochondria to provide this energy, and yet we have been deleting mitochondrial genes since our mid-twenties and thereby severely impairing the ability of our bodies to repair themselves. We must start protecting our mitochondria (the ones we have left).

---

[10] Veech RL, Chance B, Kashiwaya Y, Lardy HA, Cahill GF. Ketone bodies, potential therapeutic uses. *IUBMB Life* 2001 Apr;51:241-7.

[11] Wallace DC. Mitochondrial DNA in Aging and Disease. *Scientific American* Aug 1997.

(2)   How can we protect our mitochondria?

Dr. Douglas Wallace described how super-oxide radicals cause gene deletions and how the body has antioxidants to reduce the damage by reducing the super-oxide radicals.[11] These antioxidants included Vitamins E and C, and coenzyme Q10. The problem is when taken as pills, these antioxidants do not appear to significantly improve outcomes in most clinical trials. If we are going to improve our chances of avoiding many degenerative diseases including Alzheimer's Disease, congestive heart failure, and diabetes, we are going to have to figure out how to maintain our body's ability to produce these antioxidants and reduce oxidative stress. Burning fat as fuel rather than sugar appears to be one of those answers. As was mentioned above, burning fat as fuel helps to recycle the protective effect of vitamin E and coenzyme Q-10. Eating rare meat is an excellent source of L-carnitene, another important antioxidant and anti-aging compound. Strange as it may seem, we should avoid the symbolic apple (more sugars than are allowed in a day on the ketogenic diet).

(3)   Can we just take vitamins to prevent aging?

Nearing all of the information showing benefit from antioxidant vitamins comes from nutritional studies where people ate foods rich in antioxidants (nuts, oils, leafy vegetables). Most of the pill-based studies have shown little or no benefit. Taking large doses of one supplement may disturb the balance of vitamins and actually promote disease.

(d)   *Apoptosis (Programmed Cell Death, pronounced eh-pop-TOE-sis)*

All of our cells are programmed to last a certain time and then turn off and die. This is called apoptosis. The control of this process is complex but one switch appears to be linked to the insulin receptor. When you block the insulin-like receptor in the worm Caenorhabditis elegans, the worms live twice as long.[12] When rodents are fed low calorie diets or alternate day feedings, they also live up to twice as long.[13] [14] Insulin appears to trigger cellular processes that promote aging. Raising insulin levels accelerates most markers of aging (heart disease and cancer included) and lowering insulin action appears to slow aging (at least in the worm and rodent).[15]

So how do we reduce this programmed cell death? It is clear that patients with Type 2 diabetes, impaired glucose tolerance and insulin resistance age much faster. The good indicator of insulin resistance is the circumference of your waist. It would therefore

---

[12] Ogg WC, et al. *Nature* 1997; 389:994.

[13] Weindruch R, Walford RL. *The retardation of aging and disease by dietary restriction.* (Thomas, Springfield, IL, 1988).

[14] Bruce-Keller AJ, Umberger G, McFall R, Mattson MP. Food restriction reduces brain damage and improves behavioral outcome following excitotoxic and metabolic insults. *Ann Neurol* 1999 Jan;45:8-15.

[15] Lee C, Klopp RG, Weindruch R, Prolla TA. Gene expression profile of aging and its retardation by caloric restriction. *Science* 1999 Aug;285:1390-3.

42

appear critical to reduce the circumference of your waist by whatever means you can (short of Fen-Phen or other like drugs). You could say this is the sole purpose of this book; we must reduce our caloric intake in a healthy manner.

(e) *What Is Incomplete Carboxylation?*

Three common complications in aging include atherosclerosis (hardening of the blood vessels leading to heart disease and strokes), osteoporosis (weak bones) and Alzheimer's disease (memory loss). All three of these are worsened by incomplete carboxylation of the Gla proteins in our blood vessels, our bones and our brain.[16] This occurs because of the lack of adequate vitamin K in our diets and therefore in our tissues. The recommended daily allowance (RDA) recommended by the USDA is based on maintaining adequate blood clotting factors, which is probably one-tenth the amount required for optimal health of our blood vessels, bones and brain. The best source of vitamin K is the serious dark green leafy vegetables (see the Mediterranean Hunter-Gatherer diet below) eaten with some healthy fat (vitamin K is fat-soluble and requires fat to be absorbed).[17]

Eat your green leafy vegetables.

(f) *Allergies, inflammation, aging and cancer*

Allergies lead to inflammation of your upper and lower airways. Inflammation leads to aging and cancer. Do not take medications that control your allergy symptoms. Figure out what is promoting your allergies and get rid of it. Milk protein, sulfites in wine, peanuts, and Tartrazine (yellow dye FDA #5) promote an inflammatory reaction to dust, mold, mildew and animal dander in many individuals.[18] This also applies to allergies related to the pollen of trees and grasses. Try the Mediterranean Hunter-Gatherer diet, which eliminates most of the common triggers for allergies. If you are going to consume chocolate or other triggers, try to do it only intermittently (1-2 times per week at most).

3   Top Nine Ways to Slow Aging

(a) *Prevent or heal your diabetes or impaired glucose tolerance (insulin resistance)*

Diabetes is an excellent model of aging. The resulting glycation makes us stiff. Elevated insulin levels promote heart disease, cancer, and apoptosis (early death).

---

[16] Vermeer C, Schurgers LJ. A comprehensive review of vitamin K and vitamin K antagonists. *Hematol Oncol Clin North Am* 2000 Apr;14(2):339-353.
[17] Booth SL, Sadowski JA, Pennington JAT. Phylloquinone (vitamin K_1) content of foods in the U.S. Food and Drug Administration's Total Diet Study. *J Agric Food Chem* 1995;43:1574–9.
[18] Dixon HS. Treatment of delayed food allergy based on specific immunoglobulin G RAST testing. Otolaryngology-Head and Neck Surgery 2000 Jul:123:48-54.

(1) How do you know if this is a problem?

Look at the circumference of your waist. A waist more than 40 inches in men and 35 inches in women are considered high risk. To be less than 35 inches in men and 30 inches in women are considered acceptable, but the smaller the better. As your waist goes, so does your insulin level.

(2) Measure your insulin level.

Normal fasting insulin levels are up to 27, but anything over 10 is considered suspect for insulin resistance. A level of 5 or less is considered ideal.

(3) Measure your hemoglobin A1c.

This is the three-month diabetes test that looks at your average blood sugar. A level over 6.1% is abnormal but anything over 5.0% increases death through heart disease and cancer.[19] The same is true of your blood sugar. A level of 110 is considered normal but anything over 90 is suspect for pre-diabetes. Follow the Mediterranean Hunter-Gatherer diet to shrink your waist and make your diabetes or insulin resistance go away.

(b) *Eat the Best Foods; Avoid the Worst*

The Mediterranean Hunter-Gatherer diet is a very-low-carbohydrate diet that is rich in omega-3 oils, monounsaturated fat, green leafy vegetables, and healthy protein from fish, meat and poultry. You can eat lots of nuts and even a few berries but no grains, potatoes, or other high starch or sugar foods. Avoid excess omega-6 oils in vegetable oils.

(c) *Avoid Excess Calories*

Reduced calories but complete nutrition is associated with greater longevity. This may be an effect of low insulin levels or lower oxidative stress. The Mediterranean Hunter-Gatherer Diet is designed to keep you satisfied while lowering caloric intake.

(d) *Don't Smoke; Avoid Nitrites and Other Preservatives*

Carbon monoxide leads to excess oxidative stress. Tars lead to inflammation and chronic lung disease and cancer. Nitrites lead to inflammation of the colon, which leads to polyps and cancer.

---

[19] Khaw K, Wareham N, Luben R, Bingham S, Oakes S, Welch A, Day N. Glycated haemoglobin, diabetes, and mortality in men in Norfolk cohort of European Prospective Investigation of Cancer and Nutrition (EPIC-Norfolk). BMJ 2001 Jan;322:15-18.

(e) *Get off the Couch and Take the Stairs*

(1)　People who live in a multistory house develop fewer heart attacks (Is it the stairs or is this just a marker of more money equals better health).[20]

(2)　The greatest benefit from exercise occurs when you get off the couch and go for a walk. There is little additional benefit (other than stress reduction) from increasing this to jogging or cycling or marathon running.

(3)　In order to exercise we must avoid arthritis and other limiting illness, so take the MSM and avoid the foods associated with arthritis (corn meal in dog food is associated with arthritis in dogs- feed your dog meat).

(f) *Take just a Few Supplements*

(1)　Older rodents given chromium behave like younger rodents.[21] Could this be fooling the hypothalamus into releasing youth hormones?

(2)　Magnesium is key to bone and heart health.[22]

(3)　So is vitamin K, but get it from your green leafy vegetables.

(4)　If you don't drink fresh rainwater or eat living things, take MSM.

(g) *Avoid Allergies and other causes of Inflammation*

Do you have circles under the eyes, puffy eyes, chronic runny nose and cough, recurrent sinus infections, and fatigue? Your body is screaming at you that something is wrong. Figure it out. Milk makes more mucus in most of us. So do the sulfites in wine, wine vinegar and balsamic vinegar. Wheat irritates some people, as does chocolate (the sex surrogate).

(h) *Avoid Hostility and Depression*

Hostility releases hormones (such as angiotensin) that cause inflammation of the lining of blood vessels leading to atherosclerosis (strokes and heart attacks).[23] Depression is a manifestation of serious imbalance in your attitude and nutrition.[24] Change them both.

---

[20] Personal communication with Bernardi F.

[21] McCarty MF. Longevity effect of chromium picolinate—'rejuvenation' of hypothalamic function? Med Hypotheses 1994 Oct;43:453-65.

[22] Resnick LM. Magnesium in the pathophysiology and treatment of hypertension and diabetes mellitus. Am J Hypertens. 1997;10:368-70.

[23] Libby P, Ridker PM, Maseri A. Inflammation and Atherosclerosis. Circulation 2002 Mar;105:1135-43.

[24] Wurtman RJ, Wurtman JL. Carbohydrates and Depression. Scientific American 1989 Jan.

An example of this is the morning commute. Birds do it differently (they cooperate). If we approach the commute as a team effort, each of us trying to help the others out (and helping the people who are late the most), the world would be more pleasant and healthier (based on our lower levels of hostility hormones (angiotensin) - see Chapter 15 in Volume 2 for details).

The Best Predictor of Disease and Early Death Is the Size of Your Waist

You consume only a certain amount of food in your lifetime.

Old Chinese Proverb

3

THE CIRCUMFERENCE OF YOUR WAIST

The circumference of your waist is an excellent measure of increased fat stores and insulin resistance (particularly if combined with an elevated triglyceride level).[25] The bigger the waist, the higher the percent body fat and usually the higher the insulin level. I interpret the old Chinese proverb on the previous page to mean you can eat it now or you can eat it later, but not both. Too much food is not good your health. This effect appears to be mediated through excess insulin.

1   What is Insulin Resistance?

Insulin is one of the hormones that helps control blood sugar. It is the hormone that helps lower blood sugar by facilitating the movement of sugar into our cells. Without insulin, sugar cannot move into cells and patients can become very ill with what is called diabetic ketoacidosis. In this case only is ketosis (the burning of fat as fuel) bad for you. If you have enough insulin, ketosis (burning fat) is actually healthy (see Chapter 11 for details). Despite very high blood sugars, these patients are starving to death because of the lack of insulin. This only happens, however, in patients with Type 1 diabetes. Type 1 diabetes is associated with the destruction of the cells that release insulin.

The vast majority of patients with diabetes have Type 2 diabetes, which is caused by the body becoming resistant to the insulin so the insulin stops working. These patients are not at risk for starvation. Instead of not enough insulin, they often have very high outputs of insulin but their cells have lost their ability to respond. These patients continue to gain more weight because they lose the receptors in their brain that tells them they are satisfied. The only help for these patients is to somehow lower their insulin levels.

How do you lower your insulin level? Get rid of the carbs please! We will discuss this extensively soon. First, let's start with examining the adverse affects of insulin. Then we will look at the stories of Anna, Stephen, Gregory and Mary (below) as illustrations of many of the adverse affects of insulin.

---

[25] Depres JP; Lemieux L; Prud'homme D. Treatment of Obesity: Need to focus on high-risk abdominally obese patients. *BMJ* 2001 Mar 24; 322(7288):716-20.

2   The Adverse Effects of Insulin

(a)   *Excess insulin increases appetite making us hungry, even though we may have just eaten*

The evidence for this can be seen in any patient that is treated with excess insulin. It is impossible to lose weight if you are attempting to tightly control your diabetes using insulin. The DCCT trial[26] was a study of using intensive insulin management (versus standard care) in patients with Type 1 Diabetes. The patients in the intensive group uniformly gained weight (several kilograms each). There was a reduction in microvascular complications (problems of small blood vessels leading to kidney failure and eye disease). However, the adverse affect of hyperinsulinemia (high levels of insulin in your blood) including atherosclerosis leading to heart disease was unchanged.

(b)   *Insulin also inhibits the release of fat from fat cells, making weight loss much more difficult*

Patients with Type 2 Diabetes treated with glyburide (a medication which raises insulin levels) had significantly more weight gain compared to the metformin group (a medication which lowers insulin resistance and is associated with weight loss in most patients). The patients on glyburide also had more heart disease.[27]

(c)   *Excess insulin promotes the development of Diabetes Type 2 by increasing insulin resistance*

Increased abdominal fat leads to insulin resistance and Syndrome X resulting in Diabetes, hypertension, left ventricular hypertrophy (enlargement of your heart) and atherosclerosis (hardening of the arteries, heart attacks and strokes). Syndrome X is a constellation of problems seen in patients with insulin resistance.[28]

(d)   *Excess insulin makes you crash 1-3 hours after eating with fatigue, lethargy, decreased ability to think*

Wurtman describes the association of Seasonal Affective Disorder, Carbohydrate-Craving Obesity, and Premenstrual Syndrome.[29] Most people experience fatigue and sleepiness and become prone to committing errors after a high carbohydrate meal.

---

[26] Diabetes Control and Complications Trial (DCCT). *Am J Cardiol* (United States) May 1 1995;75(14):894-903.

[27] O'Keefe JH, Miles JM, Harris WH, Moe RM McCallister BD. Improving the adverse cardiovascular prognosis of type 2 diabetes. *Mayo Clin Proc* 1999;74:171-180.

[28] O'Keefe JH et al. Improving the Adverse Cardiovascular Prognosis of Type 2 Diabetes. *Mayo Clin Proc* 1999;74:171-180.

[29] Wurtman RJ et al. Carbohydrates and Depression. *Sci Amer* 1989 Jan; 68-75.

(e) *Excess insulin damages blood vessels and thereby promotes coronary artery disease and strokes*

Many recent reports including one by Preuss indicate that insulin resistance with hyperinsulinemia (high insulin levels) and/or hyperglycemia (high blood sugar) contribute to or even cause many chronic disorders associated with aging, i.e., chronic metabolic abnormalities including Type 2 diabetes mellitus, obesity, hypertension, cholesterol abnormalities, and atherosclerosis. [30]

In aging, similar to diabetes, the elevation in circulating glucose and other reducing sugars secondary to age-induced insulin resistance can react with proteins and nucleic acids (our genetic material) to form products that affect function and diminish tissue elasticity.

Also, adverse changes in glucose/insulin metabolism are associated with enhanced lipid peroxidation (damage to all cell membranes) secondary to greater free radical formation. Free radicals of oxygen are important known causes of tissue damage and have been associated with many aspects of aging including inflammatory diseases, cataracts, diabetes, and cardiovascular diseases. Augmented free radical formation and lipid peroxidation are not uncommon in diabetes mellitus, commonly associated with premature aging.

(f) *Excess insulin promotes the growth of cancer cells*

In a prospective study of 535 women with breast cancer, Goodwin found that the 20% of women with lowest insulin levels had 4% recurrence of their breast cancer over 7 years, while the 20% of women with highest levels had 32% recurrence. [31]

Goodwin has also shown that insulin levels are elevated in women with premenopausal breast cancer. [32] This association may reflect an underlying syndrome of insulin resistance that is independent of obesity. All results were independent of diet and other known risk factors for breast cancer. It has also been shown that metformin (a medication for diabetes that reduces insulin resistance) prevents pancreatic cancer induction in hamsters. [33] The results lend further support on the significant role of islet cells in pancreatic carcinogenesis and may explain the association between pancreatic cancer and obesity, which is usually associated with peripheral insulin resistance.

---

[30] Preuss HG. Effects of glucose/insulin perturbations on aging and chronic disorders of aging: the evidence. *J Am Coll Nutr*. 1997 Oct;16(5):397-403.

[31] Goodwin PJ et al. Insulin Resistance predicts recurrence of breast cancer. Abstract *Amer Society of Clinical Oncology*. May 2000.

[32] Goodwin PJ et al. Insulin and related factors in premenopausal breast cancer risk. *Breast Cancer Res Treat* 1998 Jan;47(2):111-20.

[33] Pour PM et al. Prevention of pancreatic cancer induction in hamsters by metformin. *Gastroenterology* 2001 Apr;120(5):1263-70.

(g) *Excess insulin promotes depression by altering brain glucose and serotonin levels*

Wurtman has described a syndrome of Carbohydrate-Craving Obesity (CCO) in which people have a disordered response to carbohydrates which impairs the effect of increased tryptophan and serotonin on the brain.[34] People with CCO report feeling refreshed and invigorated after eating carbohydrates, but the effect may take the consumption of large amounts of carbohydrates and be short-lived requiring frequent refeedings. The avoidance of simple sugars or the taking of Serotonin-raising medications appears to improve this. In one of the ongoing prospective trials of Atkin's diet, Westman has shown that not only have the subjects lost weight, 95% report more energy, 87% report less heartburn, 85% report improved mood, and 67% of women report less menstrual cramping and less premenstrual symptoms.[35]

(h) *Excess insulin speeds up the cellular clock and causes premature cell death*

Although the underlying mechanisms of aging are not understood, it is known that an insulin/IGF-signaling pathway modulates the longevity of the worm Caenorhabditis elegans.[36] The focus now is on how this pathway is regulated, how it controls nematode (the C. elegans worm) aging, and how this relates to the aging process in higher animals.[37]

3   But is this Mediterranean Hunter-Gatherer Diet the correct diet to lower insulin resistance?

(a)   *Doc, You've Got to Try The Zone*

Patients talked about the Atkins' Diet and the Zone Diet. I really wasn't interested. We (the medical establishment) used the diet based on the food pyramid (USDA approved). Then I found the preface to a book entitled The Schwarzbein Principle. The book was a summary of what a diabetes doctor had discovered listening to and working with her patients. Dr. Schwarzbein had recommended her patients eat the American Diabetes Association low-fat high-starch diet, but her patients told her after they ate a meal of pasta, bread, potatoes or rice, their blood sugars would be 50 to 100 points higher. Eating this diet required higher doses of medications, which in turn promoted weight gain,

---

[34] Wurtman RJ et al. Carbohydrates and Depression. Explores the association of Seasonal Affective Disorder, Carbohydrate-Craving Obesity, and Premenstrual Syndrome. *Sci Amer* 1989 Jan; 68-75.

[35] Eric Westman MD, Duke/Durham VA Abstract presented at the Society of General Internal Medicine in New Orleans, February 2000.

[36] Parr T. Insulin Exposure and Unifying Aging. *Gerontology* 1999, 45: 121-135.

[37] Gems D et al. Insulin/IGF signaling and aging: seeing the bigger picture. *Curr Opin Genet Dev* 2001 Jun;11(3):287-92.

which again worsened their diabetes. This was a vicious cycle, which almost invariably ended in severe vascular disease, heart attacks, strokes, and the amputation of legs.

(b)   *Those who cheat the most win?*

Perhaps the diet they were eating was making them sicker by causing their blood sugars to be higher. Dr. Schwarzbein told them to experiment with their diets and see which foods caused the least hyperglycemia (high blood sugars). The patients who cheated the most had the lowest blood sugars. These were the patients who ate bacon and eggs, steak with onions, cheese, and Brussel sprouts with mayonnaise.

(c)   *It's The Pasta, Bread, Potatoes and Rice*

Eating pasta, bread, potatoes, and rice had caused their blood sugars to rise rapidly. Eating fat and protein did not. Starch turned to sugar, which required a higher insulin level. A higher insulin level increased appetite and promoted weight gain and worsened diabetes. The high insulin level also promoted the development of atherosclerosis (heart disease, strokes, and peripheral vascular disease leading to amputations) and cancer (insulin has a growth hormone-like effect on cancer cells). And since fat does not promote the release of insulin, eating fat required much less insulin and so promoted weight loss by reducing hunger. Protein also required much less insulin, as did non-root (non-starch) vegetables.

Dr. Schwarzbein was shocked. When she looked for the clinical studies supporting the low-fat high-starch diet, she found none. All of those pretzels and pasta, bread, potatoes and rice in the AHA Prudent diet were rapidly metabolized to sugar and caused rapid insulin release. This increased hunger, weight gain, and worsening of diabetes, high cholesterol and high blood pressure. I also was shocked and disappointed in the medical establishment and the US Department of Agriculture. I decided to try *The Zone*.

(d)   *Experiment On Yourself*

First I tried it on myself. By nearly eliminating the sugar and starch from my diet, I lost 22 pounds (almost effortlessly from 166 to 144 pounds, after years of struggling with my gut). My cholesterol dropped from 210 to 160mg%. My LDL (bad cholesterol) fell from 130 to 60mg%, and my HDL (good cholesterol) rose from 72 to 91mg%! My LDL/HDL ratio was now 2/3. It seemed to work. My patients had similar experiences. I have had numerous patients lose over 50 pounds and many more lose 20 to 30 pounds. One patient's LDL cholesterol fell from 250 to 150mg%, another's from 230 to 130mg% on diet alone. My patients with diabetes have either gotten rid of their insulin injections altogether or decreased them from 70-90 units per day to 10-20 units per day, and have lost weight (and lots of it). Several patients who had recently developed Type 2 diabetes made their diabetes go away.

How do we start? Well, let's look at some examples of some successful and not so successful patients. The following five patients will illustrate the effect of excess insulin and glycation (excess sugar). See the chapters on allergy and the autoimmune response for specific examples of the adverse immune response.

(e) *Before we start, let us define some of the important parameters*

(1) Glucose: Blood sugar

Normal range is 70-110 mg%

Ideal is less than 90 mg%

(2) Hemoglobin A1c: the diabetes test

Normal range is from 3.8-6.1%.

Ideal is 5.0% or less.

Each 1% increase above 5.0% is associated with 28% more death over 4 years.[38]

Our normal range appears to still be set too high for health

Levels above 7.0% are considered very harmful, yet the average A1c of patients with diabetes in the USA is over 9.0%

(3) Cholesterol

Composed of LDL, HDL, VLDL and Triglycerides, the total cholesterol level is not as helpful as the level of each separate element.

Ideal is 160mg% unless your HDL is very high. A level of 160mg% is associated with the lowest total mortality. People with levels of 100mg% had the same mortality as people at 200mg%, the difference being the people at 100mg% had less heart disease but more cancer, homicide and suicide.

(4) LDL Cholesterol: the bad cholesterol

Levels less than 100mg% carry a low risk of heart disease. This is the goal in patients with heart disease and stroke, and patients with diabetes

Ideal is less than 80mg%.

Levels over 160mg% carry a much higher risk and medication could be considered even without heart disease or diabetes.

Levels over 190mg% should be treated with medications in most patients (except perhaps young women with no other risk factors).

---

[38] Khaw K, Wareham N, Luben R, Bingham S, Oakes S, Welch A, Day N. Glycated haemoglobin, diabetes, and mortality in men in Norfolk cohort of European Prospective Investigation of Cancer and Nutrition (EPIC-Norfolk). *BMJ* Jan 2001, 322:15-18.

(5)   HDL Cholesterol: The good cholesterol

Average for men and postmenopausal women is 45mg%.
Average for premenopausal women is 55mg%.
Ideal is greater than 55mg%.
Less than 35mg% is considered a significant risk factor.
HDL levels are suppressed by diabetes and by a low fat diet.
Olive oil, exercise and alcohol raise HDL levels.

(6)   Triglycerides: Predictor of diabetes?

Often very elevated in patients with uncontrolled diabetes.
Ideal is less than 50mg%. Less than 100mg% is good.
Part of the metabolic syndrome (Syndrome X) of diabetes, obesity, hypertension and heart disease.
Now considered an independent risk factor for heart disease.

(7)   Weight

There is no ideal weight or BMI, although a BMI of 22 or less is associated with less disease and death.[39]
A better measure is the percentage of body fat.
An easier measure is the circumference of the waist (at the umbilicus, better known as the belly button). A good waist circumference is 30-34 inches or less, depending on how tall you are.
An increase in waist circumference is associated with increased insulin resistance and Syndrome X.

(8)   Insulin

Normal range is 5-29, but any level over 10 is considered suspect for insulin resistance.
Ideal is less than or equal to 5. Less than 10 is good.

First, we'll start with Anna K:

4   Anna K: A Patient Who Made Her Insulin Resistance Go Away

Anna K is a very pleasant if somewhat anxious woman in her mid-seventies who came to me because she was feeling tired. In our first visit I looked her over. We discussed the *Staying Healthy* handout (my eight page handout discussing nutrition), then I ordered some blood tests (*We'll round up the usual suspects*) for thyroid, chemistries, blood count,

---

[39] Shaper AG; Wannamethee SG; Walker M. Body weight: implications for the prevention of coronary heart disease, stroke, and diabetes mellitus in a cohort study of middle aged men. *BMJ* 1997 May 3;314(7090):1311-7.

cholesterol panel and scheduled her to see me again after trying the lifestyle changes we had discussed.

(a)   *A Blood Sugar Of Two Hundred Eight Six!*

Her blood sugar came back alarmingly elevated at 286mg%, so I asked her to come back in sooner so we could discuss the possibility of the need for medication to help her keep her blood sugars normal. She was very resistant to the thought of taking medications. She finally agreed to take one metformin (the medication that lowers insulin resistance) in the morning. She said she was doing ok on the diet and in fact actually liked my fish stew recipe (the only patient who has ever admitted that).

She returned a few weeks later feeling much better, had lost a little weight, and was feeling very positive about where she was going with her health. Her laboratory studies are listed below:

TABLE 3-1.

	12/26/00	01/09/01	02/19/01	4/30/01	7/02/01	2/11/02
Glucose	286	100	98	96	99	108
Hemoglobin A1c	**13.0**	**10.6**	**7.4**	**6.0**	**5.7**	**5.6**
Weight	**140**	**133**	**132**	**132**	**130**	**127**

Her initial hemoglobin A1c (the 3-month average of her blood sugar) was even more alarming than initial blood sugar. A result above 7.4% is considered bad; levels above 8.4% are terrible, and above 10% you should just shoot either the doctor or the patient to get them out of their misery. Her A1c was 13.0mg%!

To give you an idea of how bad her A1c was- if your A1c rises from 6.4 to 7.4%, these is an increase in mortality (the rate of death) by 28%! The same is true from 7.4 to 8.4% and so on. Anna K's A1c of 13.0% suggested that her chance of dying over the next 5-7 years was very high.

(b)   *Her Diabetes Went Away As Soon As She Changed Her Diet*

The A1c levels dropped to normal within 4 months, which is amazing because the test measures the amount of glycation of the hemoglobin in red blood cells. Since red blood cells last 120 days, it would take at least 3 months to get rid of the old glycated blood even if her blood sugars were normal. The fact that her A1c dropped so fast means that she made her diabetes go away almost as soon as she started the diet.

(c) *Her Cholesterol Went Up and Then Back Down*

Her LDL-cholesterol levels did give me some concern, however, because a patient with Diabetes is supposed to have an LDL of less than 100mg%. Initially she was ok, but then the higher fat diet (with eggs for breakfast) made her LDL shoot up. I wanted to start her on a cholesterol-lowering medication but she refused. Fortunately the next time we checked the LDL cholesterol it was falling back to normal.

Why did her LDL go up initially? Well, simply stated, your liver makes as much cholesterol as your body needs. This is usually tightly controlled, so as you eat more cholesterol your liver makes less cholesterol (unless you are genetically programmed to make a lot of cholesterol). Insulin is one of the hormones that prompts the liver to produce more triglycerides and cholesterol. If your insulin level is too high (obesity, pre-Diabetes, or Diabetes Type 2), your liver will continue to make excess cholesterol even in the face of eating a lot of cholesterol.

TABLE 3-2.

	12/26/00	01/09/01	02/19/01	4/30/01	7/02/01	2/11/02
Cholesterol	237	240	214	210	196	197
LDL	**135**	**162**	**153**	**133**	**121**	**120**
HDL	50	54	45	58	61	61
Triglycerides	210	121	80	94	68	81
Weight	**140**	**133**	**132**	**132**	**130**	**127**

(d) *Insulin Resistance Raises Your Cholesterol and Triglycerides*

When she first came to me, Anna appeared to have significant insulin resistance and elevated insulin level. Her liver was pouring out cholesterol, but since she had followed a low fat diet (rich in sugar and starch) her cholesterol was ok. But when she got rid of sugar and starch and added a lot of cholesterol to her diet, her liver initially continued to pump out cholesterol and her LDL went significantly up. As her insulin resistance resolved and her insulin level returned to normal, her cholesterol and LDL dropped again to normal.

(e) *A New Lifestyle*

Part of what made Anna successful was her ability to adapt to a new lifestyle. A little knowledge and encouragement went a long way. Her enthusiasm and increased sense of wellbeing and energy made her into a teacher as well, helping those around her by sharing her newfound knowledge and health with the people around her.

Anna healed her Diabetes. She asked me in February if I thought it would be ok if she had an ice cream cone in July! But when it finally got to July she said she would rather feel good than eat it, so she didn't. She converted many of her employees to her new way of living and eating.

5   Gregory H: High Triglycerides and a Large Waist Equals Insulin Resistance

I had emailed Gregory the information on *Staying Healthy* and the *Diabetes Handout* even before he came to see me for the first time. He had recently developed diabetes and had started the Atkins' diet to try to make his diabetes go away.

(a)   *Making Your Diabetes Go Away*

When I first saw him I did not order blood studies because we wanted his diabetes to go away before we documented he had anything close to diabetes. I do this for patients because life insurance companies do not believe that someone can make diabetes go away. As far as they are concerned once a diabetic, always a diabetic. But that is obviously not true. Patients can make their insulin resistance resolve with simple changes in their lifestyle. It is true that most American Indians and Australian Aborigines will develop Diabetes if they eat the American Diabetes Association diet, and it will resolve on their traditional hunter-gatherer diet.

Gregory did not want to take any medications at all, but I suggested he take the chromium and magnesium because these help reduce insulin resistance. Gregory's Lab studies are as follows (he is 6' 4" tall):

TABLE 3-3.

	11/16/01	01/07/02	03/04/02	06/05/02
Glucose	125	88	85	84
Hemoglobin A1c	**9.0**	**7.0**	**6.0**	**6.0**
Weight	**310**	**292**	**284**	**290**

Note that without any medication he has brought his diabetes test (Hemoglobin A1c) down to normal. Gregory has been very successful in reversing his insulin resistance and thereby is reducing his risk of aging and disease. The goal continues to get his weight lower and his A1c into the mid-normal range.

TABLE 3-4.

	11/16/01	01/07/02	03/04/02	06/05/02
Cholesterol	212	225	181	198
LDL	**113**	**162**	**117**	**126**
HDL	34	44	43	43
Triglycerides	326	96	103	146

On the high fat diet, Gregory's initial cholesterol went up while his triglycerides fell dramatically. His HDL (good) cholesterol had also improved. As he continued to follow the diet and improve his insulin resistance, his LDL also began to improve but not quite enough. At the June 2002 office visit I finally convinced him to take a cholesterol-lowering drug to protect him until we can get his body back into shape.

6   Mary M: Unbelievable reduction in LDL; the effect of caring for self

Her results are amazing. Again her cholesterol initially went up, but as she continued the diet, her weight and diabetes continued to get better. The reduction in LDL on 3/23/2000 from 213 to 120mg% was due mostly to following the diet (I had also added 10mg of Lipitor, which might have reduced the LDL 20-40mg% at most by itself). She lost inches, her mood improved, and she was making me (the Doctor) look good by her numbers. The *Mediterranean Hunter-Gatherer Diet* had worked wonders in her.

TABLE 3-5.

	8/13/98	1/6/00	3/23/00	3/22/01	9/26/01
Cholesterol	250	317	187	230	182
LDL	**150**	**213**	**120**	**133**	**103**
HDL	62	53	40	49	46
Triglycerides	189	254	134	239	164
Weight	**170**	**166**	**163**	**159**	**154**

Her diabetes test fell to normal in January and she has continued to do well on the low carbohydrate diet.

TABLE 3-6

	8/13/98	1/6/00	3/23/00	3/22/01	9/26/01
Glucose	127	83	84	89	91
Hemoglobin A1c	**7.5**	**6.0**	**6.0**	**6.4**	**6.1**
Weight	**170**	**166**	**163**	**159**	**154**

7   John T: The Effects of Excess Glycation

(a)   *Lack of Care for Yourself*

Exhausted from doing too much for others? Are you unable to care for yourself? Do you find yourself reaching for sweets, starch, cigarettes or alcohol just to keep going? Must you complete your work, apparently no matter what the toll on your body?

- Smoking raises endorphins and adrenaline.
- So does eating chocolate and grains.
- So does drinking beer and wine (Terrific!).

I feel better already, or at least different and able to continue to slog on through what I was supposed to be doing.

- Rather than caring for myself.
- Rather than resting.
- Rather than saying: *Enough is enough.*
- Rather than saying: *That is gutenuf.*

There was a surgeon in Eden, NC who as he was finishing an operation putting in the last few sutures to close the skin (the patient was still asleep) would always say *Well, that's good enough for who it's for.* And it nearly always was.

Why can't the rest of us begin to take on that attitude? Do our best, then say out loud: *Well, that's good enough for who it's for.* Because it nearly always is.

(b)   *The Development of Pre-diabetes*

So back to the story of John T. He worked for an advertising firm, doing too much for everyone and taking on more and more duties as the need arose. He began taking care of other's needs with nothing left for him. He ate junk food at work: Tastycakes, donuts, and bagels just to have the energy to keep going. Thank goodness he didn't smoke, or he would have done that too. But he didn't need to smoke. His borderline Diabetes was all he needed. His energy began to fail; he was anxious and achy most of the time. Accidents began happening, and then…

(c)   *The Development of Heart Disease*

Chest pressure >> A very positive stress test >> Cardiac catheterization followed by the onset of unrelenting chest pain >> Emergency quadruple coronary artery bypass surgery. And that was only the beginning.

John did well through the heart operation and made it to cardiac rehabilitation. But then all hell broke loose. It was as if the dam had burst. His borderline Diabetes had evidently been silently working for years causing his tissues to become stiff and yellow.

(d)   *The Development of Diabetes and All of the Complications*

He developed the following problems in fairly short order:

- Orthostatic hypotension causing his blood pressure to drop during exercise
- Small vessel coronary disease giving him angina (chest pains) despite adequate coronary artery blood flow

- Damage to the nerves of his stomach and bladder making them sluggish and slow to empty causing intractable nausea and stomach bloating
- Numbness of his hands and feet
- And last but never least
- Erectile dysfunction (i.e. No sex!)

John had had borderline blood sugars but never met the diagnostic criteria for diabetes until mid-2000. Most of his blood sugars had been normal and his Hemoglobin A1c levels had only been above 6.5% mg% one time (the average in this country for patients with Diabetes Type 2 is around 9 mg% -normal was 4.4-6.4 mg%).

TABLE 3-7

	05/05/00	08/02/00	11/17/00	3/22/01	3/27/02	08/21/02	6/05/03
Glucose	108	143	114	76	95	78	93
Hemoglobin A1c	6.6	7.6	6.4	6.1	5.6	5.5	5.2
Weight	220	216	214	204	180	174	168

(e)   *The Incredible Impact of Self Care on Complications of Diabetes*

Up to this point, John had been a passive observer in most of his health care. I encouraged him to read *Protein Power* by Drs. Eades. He suddenly became the captain of his ship. He followed the low-carbohydrate diet to the letter. His weight dropped more than 40 pounds, his blood sugars normalized, his attitude and energy improved. He actively researched Diabetes and brought me information on many medications and supplements that he thought made sense and wanted to try. He was a new person. Well, sort of.

(f)   *Making Your Diabetes Go Away, But Too Late?*

Now John's Hemoglobin A1c levels are in the low to mid-normal range (almost as good as mine). But in some ways this is the closing of the barn door after the horse had gone. John's health was like a heavily damaged B-52 bomber plummeting 12,000 feet toward earth, the pilot and crew fighting valiantly to save their ship. Finally, seemingly only inches above the ground, they get her to level off and fly her safely back to base. But the damage has been done.

(g)   *Pre-Diabetes: The Warning Shot Across the Bow*

John's pre-Diabetes was like the warning shot across the bow of a ship. Either change direction or the next shot will be to the heart of the ship. One would like to change before you have to change. And to change before you are listing 15 degrees to starboard, and definitely before the call for abandon ship! Because that call goes up too soon as it is.

I assume if you are reading this book that you are concerned with how you feel and would like to feel better and continue to feel better. My goal is to practice medicine based not on fear of illness or death, but on self-love and self-acceptance. Gutenuf- translated *good enough*. Give yourself a break. The preceding story about John is scary, but it is not meant to put fear in our hearts. It is meant to put knowledge in our brains and strength in our souls.

(h)   *So love, not fear*

But I also think it is important to understand the risks of our behaviors. What does it mean to have a 38-inch waist when you were a 30-inch waist at age 18 years old? Is your percent body fat too high? Can you pinch an inch? It does not matter if you are big or small. The next chapter will hopefully make this clear and inspire you to greater heights (and a smaller waist).

8   Eat A Diet Rich in the Healthy Oils from Nuts, Fish, Olive Oil and Other Healthy Fats

This, however, does not mean I have eliminated carbohydrates from my diet. The Mediterranean Hunter-Gatherer diet consists of green leafy vegetables and other low-glycemic vegetables and fruit, followed by monounsaturated fat in tree nuts and olive oil, and finally the fat and protein from nuts, eggs, fish, poultry and beef.

(a)   *The Major Sources of Sugar and Starch to Avoid are as Follows:*

- Sugar, ice cream, yogurt, sorbet
- Corn syrup in sodas and syrup, baked goods and cereals
- Pasta, bread, pizza, rolls, pastries, cakes and cookies (anything made with flour)
- Root vegetables including potatoes, carrots, turnips, etc (a little is ok?)
- Rice (brown and white)- ok if you are training for a marathon (not most of us)

All of this will become perfectly clear as you see the many options of great foods in the Mediterranean Hunter-Gatherer Diet. But it is key to your success to understand the destructive effects of simple carbohydrates on your body and your sense of well being. My prediction is that as you see the reasons why bagels are death, you too will become convinced that not only do bagels promote fatigue of the body and mind, they also promote accelerated aging of your blood vessels and the rest of your body.

Eating Sugar is Death!

Eating Starch is Even Worse!

4

SUGAR AND STARCH

1   What Is Starch?

Starch is composed of glucose molecules loosely bound to each other. The digestion of starch begins at once, even in your mouth.

(a)   *Try this Experiment:*

Place two bowls on a table. Place a Saltine cracker in one bowl and chew another cracker and spit the paste into the other bowl. Place a drop of iodine in each bowl. The unchewed cracker will turn black signifying that it is starch. The chewed cracker will turn blue because it has been digested to sugar by the enzymes in your saliva. This is why we like crackers. Even sugar-free Cheerios turn to sugar in your mouth. Now eat the Special K breakfast. By the time this combination of grains, low fat milk, and orange juice gets into your small intestine you may as well have had a Coke or cake or just a cup of sugar for breakfast. Grains turn to sugar; low fat milk is mostly sugar; an orange juice is almost all sugar. You have probably already heard that a potato is equivalent to sixteen teaspoons of sugar. But potatoes are even worse than table sugar because at least the sucrose in table sugar must be absorbed and broken down from sucrose to glucose and fructose before it is free to circulate through the body as free glucose.

(b)   *How about the Glycemic Index?*

The glycemic index is a measure of how much a food will raise your blood sugar. The higher the glycemic index of a food, the higher your blood sugar (and insulin release) will be. And since we are trying to keep our blood sugar and insulin levels as low as possible, it is important to avoid the higher glycemic foods and eat the lower glycemic foods.

But you must be careful using the index, because if you add margarine to a potato the glycemic index falls but the healthfulness does not improve. This is particularly true of potato chips, which can be referred to as potato *hips* because of their ability to grow your hips (and waist).

(c) *The Glycemic Index of Common Foods*[40]

The following are examples of the glycemic index of various foods using bread as the index of 100 (rather than sugar). Our individual responses may differ from these values so keep an open mind. Some patients with diabetes report that carrots do not raise their blood sugar nearly as much as bread or dry cereals.

Glycemic index (Bread=100)

White Rice	126	Soft drink	97	Oat Bran Bread	68
Baked Potato	121	Angel Food Cake	95	Orange	62
Corn Flakes	119	Sucrose	92	Apple Juice	58
Jelly Beans	114	Cheese Pizza	86	Pumpernickel	58
Cheerios	106	Spaghetti	83	Apple	52
Carrots	101	Popcorn	79	Skim Milk	46
White Bread	101	Orange Juice	74	Black Beans	42
Wheat Bread	99	Green Peas	69	Fructose	32

Note there is not much difference between white and wheat bread, although pumpernickel is significantly less. Rice and potatoes are the worst, followed closely by the cereals (including Special K by the way) and pasta. The oils would score close to zero. Most of the nuts score in the single digits or the teens, although cashews (and peanuts) are a little higher than the others are.

(d) *So How Does One Begin To Eat Correctly?*

The Seven-Day Plan for the Mediterranean Hunter-Gatherer diet gives you a lot of options-from simple to finer foods and preparation. Much of this came from the diets of very successful patients who weren't afraid to push the envelope of what could be considered breakfast or a snack.

- Breakfast is mandatory even if it is just a handful of nuts and a tablespoon of mint or lemon flavored cod liver oil (for the omega-3 oils to help reduce depression and heart disease).
- Avoid pasta, bread, potatoes, and rice.
- Avoid all foods made from flour (unless you are crossing a desert or in a famine).
- Find a snack you like-I love nuts. Consider: vegetables and dip such as guacamole or ranch dressing made with olive oil.
- Avoid all fat free dressings and dips; these are full of corn syrup. Even Blue cheese dressing is healthier unless you're sensitive to milk products.

---

[40] Foster-Powell K, Miller JB, International Tables of Glycemic Index. *Am J Clin Nutr* 1995;62:871.

- Unsweetened chocolate or 72% pure chocolate is my treat when I am feeling suicidal.
- Very moderate use of low carbohydrate alcoholic beverages appears to be healthful.
- Avoid all fruit juices! (Yes juices!) Sugar is sugar and fruit juices are all sugar.

(e)   *So What Do You Drink? Water! Eight to Twelve Glasses Per Day!*

The rule about water is as follows:

- If you're tired, you are probably just thirsty, so drink water.
- If you're hungry, you are probably just thirsty, so drink water.
- If you're thirsty, it's too late! Your body is already dehydrated!

2   Getting Started On Living

Now stop. Visualize what we are trying to do. Sugar acts as molecular glue making our tissues stiff and yellow. Pasta, bread, potatoes and rice all rapidly convert to sugar. Eating sugar and starch causes more insulin to be released. Even whole grain bread!

This excess insulin acts as a growth factor for breast cancer, colon cancer, prostate cancer and pancreatic cancer. It also acts as a growth factor for atherosclerosis and has a growth factor for your belly, and we all know that a bigger belly promotes a higher insulin level and greater insulin resistance.

Therefore more insulin = more tumor growth, and more eating (oops-game over). So let's change directions.

(a)   *So why does the Mediterranean Hunter-Gatherer Diet work?*

Having trouble eating right? You have to learn how to cheat and get away with it. On your diet, not your spouse!

- Do you like cashews? Then eat cashews (and almonds and walnuts and Brazil nuts and pecans).
- Do you like smoked salmon? Then eat it with a fork (with capers and onions I hope).
- Do you want a beer? Then have one, but move toward a light beer such as Amstel light or better yet a Miller light, which is lower in carbohydrates. So drink but no DUI! Michelob Ultra is even lower, but it is a wheat beer that may stimulate allergies in some people (like me).
- Do you like Italian sausage? Eat it with a knife and fork with or without some eggs. But try to get the organic Italian Turkey sausage if you can, but I'm not going to argue already!

You must have food that you like, just OBLITERATE all of those bagels and muffins and donuts and cookies and cakes and French fries and chips and spaghetti and fried rice and hot dog buns and … All are death. And chips make hips that can sink ships, so watch out!

Bagels	Spaghetti
Muffins	Fried rice
Donuts	Hot dog buns
Cookies	Biscuits
Cakes Rolls	Whole wheat bread
French-fries	Crackers
Chips	

Read the list through again and visualize the cell death and tumor growth that occurs as you consume these foods. Now avoid those foods. My sixteen-year-old daughter recently told me that I have single-handedly ruined bread for her. She cannot eat it in good conscience-she is experimenting with a lower carbohydrate diet (figuring how to cheat and get away with it in her diet).

Eating sugar is death. (But a little death is OK?)

Eating starch is just like eating sugar.

Like driving your car sixty miles per hour in first gear.
Like leaving a dozen roses in the sun with no water.
Like a slow motion version of pouring gas on your body and lighting a match.

(b) ***Eating Fat and Cholesterol Does Not Make Your Cholesterol Go Up As Much As Eating Sugar***

Insulin stimulates the liver production of triglycerides and cholesterol. Insulin promotes the storage of fat in the lower stomach that supports a higher serum cholesterol level. If your insulin level is low, the more cholesterol you eat, the less cholesterol your liver makes, and vice versa. But if your insulin level is high, watch out. Your liver will continue to pour out cholesterol in addition to the cholesterol you eat. So get your insulin level down.

(c)   *Avoiding The American Heart Association Prudent Diet (the Food Pyramid diet)*

When compared to the Mediterranean diet, the American Heart Association prudent diet was associated with three times the cardiac death and six times the cancer rate.[41] The effect was so significant that the researchers felt it was unethical to continue the trial because of the much higher death rate in the low fat, high starch Heart Association diet.

The Lyon Trial

Arch Intern Med 1998 Jun 8;158(11):1181-1187.

**Mediterranean dietary pattern in a randomized trial:
prolonged survival and possible reduced cancer rate.**

de Lorgeril M, Salen P, Martin JL, Monjaud I, Boucher P, Mamelle N.
Laboratoire de Physiologie and GIP-Exercice, Centre Hospitalo-Universitaire de Saint-Etienne and School of Medicine, France.

BACKGROUND: The Mediterranean dietary pattern is thought to reduce the risk of cancer in addition to being cardioprotective. However, no trial has been conducted so far to prove this belief.

METHODS: We compared overall survival and newly diagnosed cancer rate among 605 patients with coronary heart disease randomized in the Lyon Diet Heart Study and following either a cardioprotective Mediterranean-type diet or a control diet close to the step 1 American Heart Association prudent diet.

RESULTS: During a follow-up of 4 years, there were a total of 38 deaths (24 in controls vs 14 in the experimental group), including 25 cardiac deaths (19 vs 6) and 7 cancer deaths (4 vs 3), and 24 cancers (17 vs 7). Exclusion of early cancer diagnoses (within the first 24 months after entry into the trial) left a total of 14 cancers (12 vs 2).

After adjustment for age, sex, smoking, leukocyte count, cholesterol level, and aspirin use, the reduction of risk in experimental subjects compared with control subjects was 56% (P=.03) for total deaths, 61% (P=.05) for cancers, and 56% (P=.01) for the combination of deaths and cancers. The intakes of fruits, vegetables, and cereals were significantly higher in experimental subjects, providing larger amounts of fiber and vitamin C (P<.05). The intakes of cholesterol and saturated and polyunsaturated fats were lower and those of oleic acid and omega-3 fatty acids were higher (P<.001) in experimental subjects. Plasma levels of vitamins C and E (P<.05) and omega-3 fatty acids (P<.001), measured 2 months after randomization, were higher and those of omega-6 fatty acids were lower (P<.001) in experimental subjects.

CONCLUSIONS: This randomized trial suggests that patients following a cardioprotective Mediterranean diet have a prolonged survival and may also be protected against cancer. Further studies are warranted to confirm the data and to explore the role of the different lipids and fatty acids in this protection.

---

[41] de Lorgeril M, Salen P, Martin JL, Monjaud I, Boucher P, Mamelle N. Mediterranean dietary pattern in a randomized trial: prolonged survival and possible reduced cancer rate. *Arch Intern Med* 1998 Jun 8;158(11):1181-1187.

(d) *Sure the Modern Mediterranean Diet is Better, But Don't Eat It.*

Why? Because you don't work in the fields all day, ride your bike everywhere, and you have money and access to better foods. Poor people must survive on foods that are inexpensive and accessible. Hence the dependence on pasta, breads, potatoes and milk products. Whereas these foods were the main foods available 100 years ago without the benefit of refrigeration or the trucking industry, now all of us have access to the best foods. So what are the best foods?

3 The Best Foods: The Mediterranean Hunter-Gatherer Approach

So what is this Mediterranean Hunter-Gatherer Diet anyway? My example to patients is as follows: Ok, let's say we need to cross the desert or the prairies (as many of our ancestors spent their time doing). You need to travel light and carry as many calories with as little weight as possible.

(a) *Crossing the desert*

- If you are crossing the desert, don't take broccoli!

    One pound of brocolli=100 calories
    One pound of bread = 1100 calories
    One pound of spaghetti = 2100 calories

- If you eat a pound of broccoli you get a little over 100 calories (because broccoli is mostly water and fiber), although half of the calories in broccoli do come from plant protein. Half of the carbohydrates are fiber and broccoli does reduce prostate cancer (although this is probably not a big concern in the desert).

- If I were crossing the desert I would take bread. Ready to eat, a pound of bread provides about 1,100 calories with approximately 20% from protein and a little fiber; not bad considering the circumstances.

- Spaghetti would be an even more efficient food to carry because one pound of uncooked spaghetti provides over 2,000 calories, but only about 15% from protein and very little fiber. But spaghetti must be cooked and requires water to do so, a valuable commodity in the desert.

- Lentils are high in fiber and provide about 1,000 calories per pound with 25% from protein but must be soaked and cooked, which would again slow us down.

(b) *But, we are not crossing the desert!*

So why do we choose our food this way as if we were still crossing the desert! We have ready access to all of the best foods that promote health and prevent disease, and yet we eat as though we live in the damn dessert. It does not make sense!

The cultivation of grains allowed ancient civilizations to organize into larger communities, to store and transport food to cities distant from agricultural centers, and to stockpile food to avoid famine. These grains provided valuable calories but were a poor natural substitute for the previous wide variety of foods humans consumed as hunter-gatherers.

In the 1850's it was known that a diet rich in fresh vegetables and meat was the ideal diet for a patient with diabetes, but it was felt to be unworkable because of the lack of availability (and the expense) of these foods in northern cities. This was due to the lack of refrigeration and an efficient transport system.

This is no longer true yet we continue to subsist on the foods of famine that have almost unlimited shelf life and very limited nutritional value.

French gastronome Jean Anthelme Brillat-Savarin in 1825 published in
The Physiology of Taste that he could easily identify
the cause of obesity after 30 years of listening to
one stout party after another proclaiming the joys of bread, rice
and (from a particularly stout party) potatoes.

He described the roots of obesity as a natural predisposition to consume
potatoes, grain or any kind of flour.

It appears he may have gotten it right.

Taubes G. NYTimes July 7, 2002

5

THE MEDITERRANEAN HUNTER-GATHERER DIET

1   Redefining Good Things to Eat

Now we need to re-orient our brains into accepting the fact that consuming the healthy oils in our foods is actually good for us. It is true that there are 9 calories per gram of fat and only 4 calories per gram of carbohydrates and proteins. But my experience (*and studies have shown*) that if you eliminate the starches and sugars and consume more fat you will lose weight, AS LONG AS THE CALORIES ARE ALSO REDUCED. But since fat makes you satisfied, you don't need to keep eating. My suggestion is to try the Mediterranean Hunter-Gatherer Diet and see how you feel. Most people feel terrific and lose weight (*also suggested by studies of diets of similar content presented below*).

(a)   *The Lots of Oil Diet*

- Monounsaturated fat in olive oil and almonds help to reduce LDL (bad cholesterol) and raise HDL (good cholesterol).[42] I try to consume 1-2 cups of olive oil and at least a pound of almonds and/or walnuts per week. If you are going to eat a little bread, dip it in olive oil with spices as do the people in the Mediterranean. This slows the absorption of the starch and reduces insulin response. Canola oil is OK, but not as natural as olive.

- Omega-3 oils in fatty fish (tuna, mackerel, sardines, salmon, and herring) appear to reduce both heart disease and cancer.[43] Tuna is not quite as healthy because it is lower in good fat and higher in mercury (because it is higher on the food chain, and therefore accumulates toxins). The flaxseed oil has recently been associated with increase prostate cancer, so it might be good to avoid.

(b)   *My goal for a balanced diet*

- Consume 5-15% of calories from permitted vegetables and berries (*the lesser amount if you are trying to lose weight*).

---

[42] Gumbiner B, Low CC, Reaven PD. Effects of a monounsaturated fatty acid-enriched hypocaloric diet on cardiovascular risk factors in obese patients with type 2 diabetes. *Diabetes Care* 1998 Jan; 21(1):9-15.

[43] de Lorgeril M, Salen P, Martin JL, Monjaud I, Boucher P, Mamelle N. Mediterranean dietary pattern in a randomized trial: prolonged survival and possible reduced cancer rate. *Arch Intern Med* 1998 Jun 8;158(11):1181-1187.

- A goal of 50 to 70% of calories from monounsaturated fat (*olive oil, walnuts and almonds*) and omega-3 oils in fish (*lots of liquid, healthy fat, please*).

- 15-30% of calories from protein with an emphasis on fatty fish and lean meat and poultry.

- Given the high fiber and water content of the green leafy vegetables, the diet by grams of food will contain a lot of vegetables, a lot of nuts with the moderate amounts of oils and meat, fish, eggs and poultry. Berries are acceptable but the other fruits are limited.

2   Rules of Thumb for Eating

(a)   *Eating fat makes you satisfied*

The hormone CCK that holds the food in your stomach (*making you feel full*) and tells your brain that you are satisfied is released from the first part of the small intestine in response to FAT. If you do not eat fat, you will rarely feel full or satisfied. It takes 20 minutes for CCK to be released and to get to your brain. No matter how much you eat, you will not feel satisfied for 20 minutes. Don't eat so much so quickly.

(b)   *Shop the perimeter of the grocery store; if something will not rot or sprout, don't eat it.*

(c)   *Chew each bite at least twenty times*

The food needs to be in small pieces for the body to extract the nutrients.

(d)   *Do not wash your food down with water*

Drinking lots of water while you eat dilutes the enzymes that help your body absorb nutrients. Cold water is the worst because the enzymes are much less effective at lower temperatures because they are designed to function at body temperature (approximately 98.6 degrees). But a glass or two during meals is probably ok, particularly if you are trying to lose weight).

(e)   *Don't eat pasta, bread, potatoes, or rice*

(f)   *Eat more low-glycemic vegetables and some fruit (see below for how to do this)*

(g)   *Eat some protein and good fat with every meal and snack (almonds and walnuts are an excellent choice)*

(h)   *How About the Drinking of Alcohol?*

Non-sweetened alcoholic beverages appear to reduce blood sugar and insulin levels and reduce heart disease. Alcohol appears to be metabolized as liquid fat, not as sugar (as is seen when a person with diabetes consumes alcohol; their blood falls rather than rising). But not recommended for everyone due to the ever-present risk of alcoholism. Limit to 14/week for men, 9/week for women. See more on Alcohol in Chapter Fourteen.

3   Evidence for the rich in oil Mediterranean Hunter-Gatherer Diet

(a)   *You can lose weight and improve your health eating 50-70% of your calories as fat*

James Hays MD[44] did a study which included 187 patients with Diabetes type 2 (84 men, 73 women). During the first year the subjects ate the American Diabetes Association diet. The second year they followed a higher fat diet. The ADA diet had 1800 calories with 30% fat, 50% carbohydrate and 20% protein. The high fat diet was 1800 calories with 50% fat, 20% carbohydrate and 30% protein (fat 90% saturated, 10% monounsaturated similar to the Atkin's diet).

Results: Average weight loss: 40 pounds; LDL: 133 fell to 105; HDL: 44 rose to 47; Triglycerides: 229 declined to 182; 90% of patients achieved ADA targets for HbA1c, HDL, LDL, and triglycerides.

(b)   *A high fat meal raises your insulin level less than a high protein meal*

TK Nordt and colleagues demonstrated that insulin levels increased after the protein-rich meal but decreased after a fat-rich meal.[45] The article was entitled *Influence of breakfasts with different nutrient contents on glucose, c peptide, insulin, glucagon, triglycerides, and GIP in NIDDM.* The study groups ate three different breakfasts varying in the amount of fat and protein (group 1) or only in fat (group 2).

(c)   *Polycystic Ovary Syndrome improves on a 50% fat diet*

Polycystic Ovary Syndrome (PCOS) appears to be mediated by insulin resistance. Hays did a study demonstrating that significant weight loss was associated with lower fasting insulin/glucose ratios and lower serum triglycerides.[46] Three of 8 women desiring pregnancy became pregnant; 3 of 4 women reported mild to moderate subjective

---

[44] Hays J. A higher fat diet promoted improvement in all parameters of Diabetes control. *Abstract presented at the Endocrine Society 82nd Annual Meeting,* May 2000.

[45] Nordt TK; Besenthal I; Eggstein M; Jakober B. Influence of breakfasts with different nutrient contents on glucose, C peptide, insulin, glucagon, triglycerides, and GIP in non-insulin-dependent diabetics. *Am J Clin Nutr* 1991 Jan;53(1):155-60.

[46] Hays J. Carbohydrate Restricted High-Fat Non-Ketotic Diet Improves Polycystic Ovary Syndrome. *Abstract presented at the Endocrine Society 82nd Annual Meeting.* May 2000.

improvement of excess facial hair; 7 of 8 women reported return of regular menstrual periods. The diet used was again 50% fat, 20% carbohydrates and 30% protein.

(d)   *If you cannot afford beans, then eat bread!*

DJ Jenkins showed that bread gives a much higher glycemic response than beans.[47] *(But if you can afford low starch vegetables, olive oil, fish, meat, nuts and berries, eat them.)*

(e)   *It appears prudent to avoid the use of the ADA diet (low-fat, high-carbohydrate diets containing moderate amounts of sucrose) in patients with Type 2 diabetes.*

Coulston described the deleterious metabolic effects of high-carbohydrate, sucrose containing diets in patients with non-insulin dependent diabetes mellitus (this was the recommended ADA diet).[48] Two test diets consumed in random order over 15 days each: ADA diet containing 20% protein, 20% fat, and 60% carbohydrate with 10% of calories as sucrose; the higher fat diet containing 20% protein, 40% fat, and 40% carbohydrate with 3% of calories as sucrose.

Incremental glucose and insulin responses from 8am to 4pm were significantly higher with the ADA diet and 24 hour urine glucose excretion was significantly higher (*55 versus 26grams/24hr*) with the ADA diet. HDL concentrations dropped with the ADA diet *(HDL is the good cholesterol, so the lower level was worse for the patient).* LDL concentrations did not change on either diet.

(f)   *Eating almonds, walnuts, cashews, pecans (and even peanuts?) appears to protect against heart attacks*

Sabate stated that perhaps one of the most unexpected and novel findings in nutritional epidemiology in the past 5 years has been that nut consumption seems to protect against heart attacks. In a large, prospective epidemiologic study of Seventh-day Adventists in California, Sabete found that the frequency of nut consumption had a substantial and highly significant inverse association with risk of heart attacks and death.

---

[47] Jenkins DJ: Glycemic Responses to Food in non-insulin dependent diabetes *Am J Clin Nutr* 1984 Nov;40(5):971-81.
[48] *Am J Med* 1987 Feb;82(2):213-20.

(g) *Eating nuts is associated with increased longevity*

The Iowa Women's Health Study and other studies[49] also documented an association between nut consumption and decreased risk of IHD. The protective effect of nuts on IHD has been found in men and women and in the elderly. Importantly, nuts have similar associations in both vegetarians and non-vegetarians. The protective effect of nut consumption on IHD is not offset by increased mortality from other causes. Moreover, frequency of nut consumption has been found to be inversely related to all-cause mortality in several population groups such as whites, blacks, and the elderly. Conclusion: Nut consumption may not only offer protection against IHD, but also increase longevity.

4   What to Eat

So you want to know exactly what to eat. The following is a partial list of foods. Chapter Seven will give a more complete presentation of suggestions and recipes to help you get started. If I were truly smart, I would move to the south of France or the north of Italy where all of the best foods flourish in the perfect weather.

(a) *Vegetables*

(1) Best: broccoli, cauliflower, Brussel sprouts, artichokes, celery, leeks, asparagus, endive, rhubarb, parsley, garlic and other spices, greens of collard, mustard, kale, cabbage, kohlrabi and lettuce, okra, Dandelion greens, escarole, horseradish, seaweed, Swiss chard, etc.

(2) *Acceptable*: carrots, onions, spinach (very high in oxalates), mushrooms, turnips.

(3) *Limit:* Brown rice, Yams.

(4) Avoid: Baked potatoes, potato chips, mashed potatoes, pretzels and all wheat products.

(b) *Oils*

(1) Best: Olive oil-extra virgin, olive oil-light, tree nut oils (almond, walnut), grape seed oil, fish oils.

(2) Acceptable: butter, high oleic safflower oil.

(3) Limit: Canola oil (too processed?), peanut oil.

(4) Avoid: Soybean oil, corn oil, partially hydrogenated oils.

---

[49] Hu FB; Stampfer MJ Nut consumption and risk of coronary heart disease: a review of epidemiologic evidence. *Curr Atheroscler Rep* 1999 Nov;1(3):204-9.

(c) *Meats   (All range fed without hormones or antibiotics).*

(1) Best: Eggs and meat from chickens raised without hormones or antibiotics, turkey, organic beef, range-fed or wild venison, duck, buffalo, goose, rabbit, moose, elk.

(2) Acceptable: Conventionally raised turkey (they tend to die if raised with too many hormones and antibiotics).

(3) Limit: Conventionally raised (mass produced using hormones and antibiotics) poultry, eggs, beef, etc.

(4) Avoid: Conventionally raised pork.

(d) *Fish   (Most fish are excellent sources of protein and omega-3 oils).*

(1) Best: Salmon, sardines, bass, trout, squid, whitefish.

(2) Acceptable: These fish are higher in mercury and other toxins so avoid the dark meat tuna, swordfish, especially for children and women of childbearing age.

(3) Limit: These are scavengers and may be contaminated with pathogenic bacteria so choose carefully. Oysters, clams, mussels, and lobster.

(4) Avoid: Certain fish are endangered and should be allowed to recover. Orange Roughie, Striped Bass.

(e) *Nuts and seeds*

(1) Best: almonds, walnuts, Brazil, pecans, macadamia, acorns, hickory, filberts, sesame, coriander, celery, anise, caraway, cumin, dill, fennel, mustard, pumpkin, and any others edible raw.

(2) Acceptable: cashews (I usually buy roasted/salted cashew pieces because they already are not that good for you, and mix them in with the unroasted nuts), pistachios, sunflower seeds.

(3) Limit: peanuts, soy nuts (actually beans).

(f) *Fruits   (Avoid all but the "Best" while you are trying to lose weight)*

(1) Best: cucumbers, avocados, olives, zucchini, tomatoes, etc.

(2) Acceptable: apples, apricots, cherries, papaya, pineapple, plums.

(3) Limit: bananas, watermelon, cantaloupe, oranges, lemons, limes, tangerines, pears, peaches, melons, plums, prunes, dates, mango (unless you are allergic).

(4) Avoid: all commercial fruit juices.

(g) *Berries*

> *(1) Best:* organic blueberries, raspberries, blackberries, strawberries are best, but wash them carefully. These are lower in sugar and higher in fiber.

> *(2) Acceptable:* conventional blueberries, raspberries, blackberries, and strawberries, but again wash them carefully due to the pesticides.

> *(3) Limit:* currants, grapes and all dried fruit that are higher in sugar.

Note: People with arthritis may want to avoid the nightshade vegetables to see if it improves their arthritis: tomatoes, peppers, eggplant, and potatoes.

5   What not to eat: The Foods of Famine

These are the foods that can be stored for long periods of time and are referred to as the products of civilization. They allowed us to gather in communities and survive living in climates with a short growing season. But although they provide calories, they are very short in important nutrients that prevent illness and optimize health. So avoid them when you can.

(If you can not eat it raw, then don't eat it.)
If even mold or bacteria won't eat it, then you don't eat it either.

(a) *Grains*   *(See Chapter Thirteen- What's Wrong with Wheat)*

> *(1) Worst:* all grains, especially corn and wheat that also promote allergies.

> *(2) Acceptable:* rolled oats and rice are usually ok, but I still try to get my calories from vegetables, nuts and healthy oils. Non-wheat beers are ok unless you have Gluten-sensitive enteropathy (Celiac Sprue).

(b) *Potatoes and other root vegetables*

> *(1) Worst:* all varieties of potato turn rapidly to sugar in your body so avoid them. Especially bad are all French fries and potato chips that contain cancer-forming chemicals.

> *(2) Acceptable:* Small amounts of yams, garlic, onions, beets, turnips, etc. are ok but still not as good as the green leafy vegetables.

(c) *Dairy*   *(See Chapter Twelve- Reasons to Avoid Cow's Milk)*

> *(1) Worst:* all cows' milk, cheese, yogurt, whey, casein, and all products made with them.

> *(2) Acceptable:* goat's milk and cheese (Feta cheese) and sheep milk products. The protein in cow's milk is the problem, so the use of a little butter or heavy cream is ok (very low in casein).

(d) *Sugar*

(1) Worst: fructose, sucrose, maltose, dextrose, lactose, corn syrup and sweeteners, molasses, and all products made from them. This includes processed *fruit juices* (these are mostly sugar; you may as well have a Coke with a vitamin C tablet).

(2) Acceptable: a Tsp. of sugar in your coffee or tea will not kill you (only 4-5 grams of sugar). In comparison, a 12-ounce soda has 8 Tsp. of sugar (equivalent to a medium-sized potato!).

(e) *Bad oils and fat*

(1) Worst: The omega 6 oils (corn, safflower, sunflower, Crisco, soybean and vegetable oil) may promote cancer and should be avoided, as well as the partially hydrogenated vegetable oils.

(2) Acceptable: a little peanut oil (as in Chinese food) is ok, as is the high oleic safflower and sunflower oils.

(f) *Beans*

(1) Worst: Pinto and Navy contain lignans that may promote an abnormal immune response. Lima, wax, fava beans, and all products made from them (see section of The Other Side of Soy).

(2) Acceptable: You may include some hard beans (like black beans, etc.) which have a much lower glycemic index compared to the others. Peas, peanuts, and pure chocolate (cocoa butter has been associated with reduced heart disease) are also ok in limited amounts unless you are allergic.

The Most Common Mistakes

1. Eating too much fruit- especially the high sugar fruits like bananas, apples, melons, and citrus.
2. Drinking fruit juices like orange juice- these are full of sugar!
3. Having cereal with low fat milk for breakfast- this is all simple carbohydrates. You can get your fiber and calcium in healthier forms.
4. Eating too many nuts. Measure the amount of nuts to put in your baggy for snacks. You can have 1-2 oz if you are trying to lose weight or 3-5 oz if you are maintaining your weight.
5. Not drinking enough water- leading to constipation. Your body will steal the water it needs from the colon to run the body, leaving you constipated.
6. Not taking the Magnesium, chromium, and MSM (see Chapter 10 on nutritional supplements)- leading to constipation. Most of my patients have 1-3 bowel movements per day. If you are not, take Magnesium 500mg 1-2 tabs twice daily, MSM 3,000 mg in the morning and chromium picolinate 500 mcg in the morning. And drink your 8 glasses of water per day minimum.
7. Cheating too much- see next page.

The Ways I Cheat *(and frequently!)*

1. Decaffeinated coffee/ or 100% pure cocoa (sometimes real coffee as well)
2. 73% or (better) 99% pure chocolate bars (baker's chocolate-unless you are allergic!)
3. Roasted and salted cashews in with my unroasted unsalted mixed nuts
4. Miller Lite 1-3 per day
5. I do much of my exercise/weight lifting/stretching lying down
6. Feta goat cheese is usually fine (goat's milk does not cause as much allergic reaction)
7. I eat sausage (usually the organic Italian turkey sausage from the organic food market)
8. I eat bacon (usually organic turkey bacon from the organic foods market)
9. I eat poached eggs or sunny side up (exposing the egg yolk to heat and oxygen oxidizes the cholesterol- such as happens when you scramble eggs!)
10. If you are good 95% of the time, a little cheating doesn't seem to catch up with you, but it is a slippery slope to failure if you stray to wheat or milk products.

If your belt is getting tight, you are cheating too much- Retreat!

6

GETTING READY FOR THE FIRST WEEK

Don't think fat grams! Don't think calories!

Think:
What is this food doing to my blood sugar and insulin level? !

1   Nutrition for Women *(Men, Add Fifty Percent Please)*

If you eat something that is mostly sugar or starch, your blood sugar will rise rapidly requiring a much higher insulin level. This excess insulin promotes weight gain, diabetes, heart disease, cancer, depression, (not to mention fatigue and cravings) and early death The excess sugar acts like molecular glue (glycation) turning your organs yellow and hard (the hallmarks of aging).

But if you are going to be successful reducing sugar and starch, you will not only need to change your attitude but also your environment. You must surround yourself with foods you enjoy which are lower in sugar and you must add more healthy oils to satisfy your appetite and cravings. Some of these food suggestions may seem crazy but they appear to work well in clinical practice (and life). So here goes.

(a)   *Getting Ready*

Giving up sugar and starch is similar to quitting smoking. I've heard you do it not because you really want to, but because you don't feel terrific or your children are making fun of you. It is never easy to quit consuming a substance. But then you discover you feel better (and free from the craving noose around your neck). After a while you decide you would never go back. You cheat and you find out you don't feel as well. You just feel off. These reactions confirm that the changes you made are working.

You will need to clean house of temptations including all baked goods, ice cream, **and** anything not listed that may pull you off your path. It is similar to putting away

83

ashtrays and other cues for smoking. This approach is designed to offer you satisfaction with little forethought and effort on your part. Just have some nuts or open the refrigerator to find something you like (that is also good for you). You will also need to busy yourself with other activities besides eating- such as exercise!

I suggest you try a couple of the supplements. The only ones that make you feel better are the chromium (better mood) and MSM (less aches and pains of getting older). The omega-3 oils in fatty fish do reduce cardiac arrhythmias (extra beats of the heart) and also makes me a nicer person (I now apologize to my wife after I am mean to her; well, most of the time). All of the others just fill in the blanks of our diets and I consider very optional if you are eating well.

I have included grocery lists of foods and supplements to purchase before starting. This will include two different approaches- the *Price is no object for health* approach and the *More cost-effective* approach. We will start with the *Price is no object* approach.

I suggest shopping for the produce and meat/fish on Sunday so you will be ready for the week. You will buy produce for one week and nuts and vitamins for one month, so the costs shown will average out over that time-span.

You will need to visit the following stores:

(1) Your local nut store (or online)
(2) Your local vitamin store (or online)
(3) Your local organic food store for organic produce, fruits, and meat/fish/poultry
(4) Your local grocery for less expensive staples

(b)   *Buying Fresh versus Frozen*

I agree with those who say eating fresh food is better (ideally vegetables from your garden, eggs from your chickens, fish caught from your boat, and meat that you hunted), but my wife won't let me have chickens. You lose nutrients when you store, freeze, or dry food (you also lose nutrients when you cook foods, so nothing is perfect). If I have the time I prefer growing or buying fresh food.

Freezing or storing food does decrease the nutritional content by half or more (give or take). So I eat twice (or more) as many green leafy things (especially if they have been frozen). And this is easy to do because the vegetables are already cut-up and placed in handy bags or boxes in my freezer. It is mighty convenient to open the freezer, take out a bag of good frozen vegetables and heat them in a little water. Then remove from heat and add some olive oil and garlic. This is, of course, after you have defrosted the fish, chicken, or meat and broiled/sautéed/stewed/ baked it for a quick available dinner. Sometimes I make frozen Brussel sprouts and assorted greens heated in olive oil with garlic and pepper for a quick snack (or with Tamari sauce or soy sauce).

2   The Money is No Object Approach

Ideally we would go (on a daily basis) to the local fresh market and buy fresh fish, broccoli, salad greens, red peppers, zucchini, and fruit and eat as much raw as possible. Prepare with lots of olive oil to encourage the absorption of fat-soluble nutrients. But life is full of compromises (I still by frozen berries and frozen leafy vegetables).

So let's go shopping...   **Shopping lists**

(a)   ***The Nut Store***

Nuts for the First Month: (and each month thereafter)
Your local nut house or online; (buy in bulk, it is usually cheaper). I buy six pounds of each (with two of us eating, except Brazil nuts). Try to find organic nuts if you can.

(1)	3 lbs. unsalted raw almonds	11.50
(2)	3 lbs. unsalted raw walnuts	12.00
(3)	3 lbs. salted cashew pieces (roasted)	9.75
(4)	3 lbs. raw Brazil nuts	8.25
(5)	1 lb. raw macadamia nuts (optional, 9.99)	

Total: 40.50

(74.00 for two people)

(b)   ***The Vitamin Store***

Supplements for Three Months:

(1) Chromium polynicotinate 200mcg, (1/day) 10.00
(2) Magnesium citrate 250mg, 90 caps (1-2/day) 5.00
(3) Calcium 500mg with Vitamin D (1-2/day) 10.00
(4) MSM 1000mg, 150 caps (3/day) 30.00
(5) One Daily without iron (1/day) 12.00
(6) Cod liver oil, 16 oz (1 Tbs./day) 12.00 (buy fresh each month)

Total: 79.50

(c)   *The Local Grocery Store for the Basics*

Daily Staples: (approximately one-month supply, or more)

(1) Olive oil- light, full bodied,	12.00	(for cooking)
(2) Olive oil- extra virgin,	20.00	(for dressings)
(3) Rice vinegar (don't worry; it's good)	3.00	
(4) Garlic cloves (3 cloves)	2.00	
(5) Dried Basil (or from the garden?)	2.00	
(6) Dried Parsley (or from the garden?)	2.00	
(7) Dried Fennel (or from the garden?)	3.00	
(8) Ginger powder	3.00	
(9) Red and black pepper	1.00	
(10) Morton's Lite Salt	2.00	
(11) Cans of tuna (albacore) five cans	7.50	
(12) Cans of salmon (small cans) three cans	4.50	
Total:	62.00	

(d)   *The Kitchen Store*

(1) Garlic press (fresh pressed garlic has anti-viral, anti-bacterial, and anti-fungal activity, as well as boosting the immune system)
(2) Stainless steel pots and pans with lids (no aluminum, please)
(3) Colander
(4) Egg poacher (usually holds three eggs)
(5) Egg coddlers- usually porcelain from Great Britain (optional)
(6) A blender
(7) A food scale (to quickly measure your nuts and other items)
(8) Measuring spoons

(e)   *The Kitchen Garden*

If you have any sunny area in your yard or neighborhood (most people won't steal what you are going to plant), you can grow the following vegetables and spices with almost no work on your part. You can plant seedlings from your local nursery in the spring. Many of these will winter over in states below NY. The mulch I use is the bags of leaves neighbors leave by the street. I grind the leaves with my lawn mower to make mulch.

(1) Kale (grows like a weed with no care- just mulch well so you don't have to weed)

(2) Collards (same as kale, may grow these together. The tender new leaves are good eaten raw)

(3) Arugula (a somewhat bitter green that grows well; again, mulch well)

(4) Parsley and Italian parsley

(5) Fennel (tastes like licorice, even my son likes it)

(6) Basil (will not survive frost- harvest before first frost. You can make pesto and freeze it, or dry by hanging in the kitchen, then place in dry container)

(7) Broccoli

(8) Brussel sprouts

Frozen Pesto:

Harvest your basil plants prior to the first frost. Collect the leaves, wash well and place in blender with ½ cup of olive oil per 2 packed cups of leaves. Blend until smooth. Add 1 Tbs. of Parmesan cheese and 1/3 cup almonds for each ½ cup of olive oil you have added. Blend until smooth and then decant into ice cube trays and freeze overnight. In the morning, remove pesto from trays and place in a freezer bag. You will now have pesto for the winter.

(f) *The Organic Food Market*

Vegetables and fruit: Shop frequently so perishables will stay fresh
(I often buy frozen because they keep longer, for those of us who get to the store infrequently)
(Fresh is not really fresh; it has usually been sitting around for days or weeks?)

(1) Soy sauce (no sugar or preservatives)	3.00
(2) Grape seed oil mayonnaise	3.50
(3) Spinach, fresh or frozen, 16 oz	1.75
(4) Turnip greens, fresh or frozen, 16 oz	1.50
(5) Broccoli flowerets, fresh or frozen, 16 oz	1.75
(6) Brussel sprouts, fresh or frozen, 16 oz	2.25
(7) Fresh asparagus, 1 bundle	3.00
(8) Celery, 1 head	2.00
(9) Carrots, small, bag, 8 oz	1.50
(10) Strawberries, fresh or frozen, 16 oz	2.30
(11) Blueberries, fresh or frozen, 16 oz	2.80
(12) Raspberries, fresh or frozen, 16 oz	3.00
Total	28.00

Meat/Poultry/Fish

(1) Haddock fillets, 16 oz		8.00
(2) Turkey bacon, 12 oz		4.00 (optional)
(3) Smoked salmon-no nitrites, 4 oz		5.00
(4) Cold water shrimp (frozen), 12 oz		6.00
(5) Scallops (frozen), 6 oz		4.00
(6) Crabmeat (canned), 6 oz		3.00
(7) Chicken breast, 8 oz		3.00
(8) Organic beef, 6 oz	3.00	
	Total:	36.00

3. Give Us This Day Our Daily Fish And Vegetables

We are now ready to begin. In the following chapter are suggestions for three meals, a snack and a dessert. Eat as much as you feel good eating. The snacks are there if you get hungry after eating your salads, etc. But the snacks are not required.

(a) *Breakfast, however, is required.*

Even if it is just the tablespoon of mint-flavored cod liver oil, the supplements, and a few nuts. If you do not eat in the morning (breaks your overnight fast), your body will assume there is inadequate food available and will slow your metabolic rate. This slower metabolic rate makes it much harder to lose weight and can make you feel sluggish and less like exercising. But your breakfast must have some healthy fat and protein as listed below.

(b) *Eating oil and fat makes you satisfied.*

If you are hungry during the day (or night), eat a little healthy fat (like nuts or nut-butter) and then go for a walk (to give the food time to work). Add olive oil to all vegetables to improve absorption of fat-soluble nutrients. Fat causes your intestine to release cholecystekinin (the hormone that tells your brain you have eaten). You will not feel satisfied after eating, NO MATTER HOW MUCH YOU EAT, until you eat some fat. The cholecystekinin takes 15-20 minutes to work so be patient and eat slowly.

(c) *Coffee is ok, but green tea is better?*

Caffeine is ok as long as you do not have heartburn, esophageal reflux, palpitations, or breast cysts. Caffeine increases frequency of bowel movements and therefore probably reduces colon cancer, and coffee makes you think faster (but not smarter?). On the downside, coffee does leech calcium from your bones and raise your insulin levels, so don't overdo. I try to drink decaffeinated coffee most of the time (3% caffeine as opposed to the 7% caffeine of regular coffee). Is this similar to drinking light beer?

(d)   *What about Alcohol?*

Alcohol has been shown to reduce blood sugar and insulin levels (these are both good things) and is associated with a higher HDL (good) cholesterol. The alcohol appears to be metabolized as liquid fat and so does not raise your blood sugar but can actually lower blood sugar and insulin levels. People with diabetes will need to reduce or stop their insulin or other diabetes medication if they take a drink. Alcohol in excess (see below) is associated with liver disease (fatty liver and cirrhosis), heart disease (irregular beats of the heart), brain disease (depression, dementia, and neuropathy) and social ills (auto accidents, poor inter-personal relationships, and alcoholism). Avoid alcohol if you have any of the alcohol-related problems or hepatitis C. See chapter fourteen for more details about alcohol consumption.

Those who do not drink alcohol do not need to start drinking alcohol.

The Definition of Moderate Drinking
These are limits, not goals please!
Women: 1-2/day, max 9/wk.
Men: 1-3/day, max 14/wk

(e)   *Nutritional Supplements*

(1) Chromium polynicotinate 200mcg	1 in the morning
(2) MSM 1000mg	3-4 in the morning
(3) Magnesium citrate 250mg	1-2 per day
(4) Calcium citrate 500mg with vit D	1-2 per day
(5) Cod liver oil	1 Tbs. in the morning

Optional
(1) (Coenzyme Q-10 75mg)	1 in the morning
(2) (Alpha Lipoic Acid 300mg)	1 in the morning

(f)   *The Eating Suggestions*

You will find the nutritional content of the food you are eating listed. This is provided to give you an idea of what you are doing, not so that you can obsess over numbers of calories or fat grams. You will also find that many of your calories are coming from the healthy oils. Although oils are very rich foods (nine calories per gram versus four calories for protein and carbohydrate), avoiding the starches and sugars allow you to consume such high-caloric foods as nuts and avocados without gaining weight.

(g)   *Fiber does not count as usable carbohydrates*

It is not that dietary fiber is not important. It is key to try to consume at least 20 grams of fiber per day as well as drinking your eight to twelve glasses of water per day to keep your bowels regular. But it is true that fiber does not count in terms of raising your insulin level. In fact, you must subtract the fiber grams from the total carbohydrate grams to get the usable carbohydrates. As you will see….

(h)   *The Seven Day Plan For Women Is Different From The Seven Day Plan For Men*

One of my patients observed that if 50% of my patients had a particular issue I would write something to address it. And yet, she complained the original 7-day plan was written specifically for men. I admitted I had based the diet on how I eat, and since I am a man it closely resembles how a man can eat to feel good and lose weight. But in order for women to lose weight, they need to consume fewer calories than men as outlined in nutrition for women.

**THE MEDITERRANEAN HUNTER-GATHERER
NUTRITION FOR WOMEN
SEVEN DAY PLAN**

Better Known As:

The Sexy Long-Life Eating Plan

The Seven Day Plan
Is
A Life Long Eating Plan

(Not just for 7 days!)

1   A High Oil Diet Reduces Appetite, Muscle Loss, and the Markers of Aging

So we have discussed how eating fat and oils releases cholecystekinin, a hormone which suppresses appetite. A high oil diet also does the following:

- Promotes ketosis, which suppresses appetite
- Ketones are an excellent source of energy for muscles and the brain (see Chapter 11 Ultimate Sports Nutrition)
- Ketones reduce oxidative stress and slow aging
- Ketones improve Co-enzyme Q-10 levels which is associated with less Alzheimer's disease
- It is important to continue the ketosis from an overnight fast by minimizing carbohydrates for breakfast

(a)   *Therefore, Eating Sugar is Death.*

And eating starch is even worse. Especially if you consume sugar and starch for breakfast. Try to save your carbohydrates for the evening hours, which will help induce restful sleep without adversely affecting daytime energy consumption or insulin release. Who cares if you get hungry while you sleep, as long as you don't wake up!

(b) *Ketosis Appears To Be A Good Thing*

The hunter-gatherer probably spent much of his or her life in ketosis while hunting and gathering for food. Is this the Atkins' diet? No and yes. Dr. Atkins' diet is a ketogenic diet but includes foods that are known to be unhealthy. This includes the nitrites and other preservatives in cured meats, as well as the hormones and antibiotics often used in the production of conventional meat, poultry and farm-raised fish. In addition, the over-consumption of certain vegetable oils (high in Omega-6 oils) may promote the growth of tumors.

2 Nutrition for Women: The New Seven-Day Plan

(a) *Weight Loss Diet for Women (Men add 50% more food per serving)*

Why is this called Nutrition for Women? Because the first plan I created was based on how my successful patients (all men) and I had eaten. But my female patients complained that they were not losing weight nearly as fast (this is also true of the Atkins' Diet that contains too many calories for women). The original plan I set forward was based on 1800 calories per day and no women (except athletes) will lose weight eating that much. So I was requested to create a plan specifically for women. Men need only to eat half again as much (50% more) than their female counterpart.

    (1) Calories:1000-1200 Calories per day
    (2) Fat: 60-70%; 80-100 grams per day (720-900 calories)
    (3) Carbohydrate: 7-10%; 20-30 grams per day (80-120 calories)
    (4) Protein: 20-30%; 60-90 grams per day (240-360 calories)

Men: Increase each serving size by ½ (50% more) and you will still lose weight. Examples include the following:

Eggs: have 2 or 3 instead of 1 or 2 (one whole egg and one egg white if cholesterol is high)
Meat, fish, and poultry: 3 ounces instead of 2 for breakfast
6 ounces instead of 4 for lunch
9 ounces instead of 6 for dinner

(b)   *Maintenance Diet For Women*

       (1) Calories: 1500-1800 Calories per day

       (2) Fat: 50-60%; 80-100 grams per day (720-900 calories)

       (3) Carbohydrate: 15-20%; 50-75 grams per day (200-300 calories)

       (4) Protein: 15-25%; 60-90 grams per day (240-360 calories)

       (5) Women may increase most serving sizes by 50%

       (6) Men may increase some serving sizes of their choice by 100%

       (7) Both should add some fruit and more vegetables; but keep the digestible carbohydrates (total minus fiber) to less than 30 grams (for women) and 40 grams (for men).

3   Guidelines for Healthy Eating

(a)   *Best is Better Than Better, Which is Better Than Good*

You may mix and match from each column (Best, Better and Good) on the following pages (see the tables below and this will become clearer). An example is choosing the salmon for breakfast but having real coffee instead of the Organic Italian turkey sausage with green tea (I usually choose the decaf if I have the option although I like green tea also). Brewed decaf coffee has 40% of the caffeine of regular coffee, so if you get the large you come out even.

(b)   *Buy Good Foods*

Try to buy all organic meats and poultry and wild (not farm raised) fish. Do not eat farm-raised salmon; look for wild salmon at your organic food market. Tuna, swordfish and other large predator fish have higher levels of mercury and other toxins. The white Albacore tuna is better because most of the toxins are concentrated in the darker fatty part of the fish (less in the white part of the fish).

(c)   *Eat Some Nuts*

Put the nuts (your snack) into a baggie to carry with you in case you get hungry (being prepared prevents failures). There is always a donut shop nearby (I call this Donut Death) so be prepared to eat in a healthy way. Most of the nuts I eat are unroasted and unsalted; but I like roasted and salted macadamias and cashews as a treat (but cashews are much higher in simple carbohydrates).

(d)   *Balance Your Omega 6 and Omega 3 oils*

When you begin to eat a lot more oils and fats, it is important to make sure you are not consuming too much of the omega 6 oils. These are present in the vegetable oils and in nuts. This is why I encourage you to eat the fatty fish, including the salmon, herring, sardines and mackerel. The cod liver oils are also excellent sources of omega 3 oils. Some other options include the grape seed oil mayonnaise (Vegennaise), which tastes a lot like real mayonnaise but without the soybean oil. Using butter or olive oil increases the monounsaturated fats and avoids the polyunsaturated fats.

(e)   *Worrying About Cholesterol*

If you have diabetes or high cholesterol based on a family trait of excess cholesterol production, I suggest you avoid excess dietary cholesterol (eggs, sardines, shrimp, lobster, and fatty steak). The kippered herring is ok, as are the whites of eggs (only the yolk contains cholesterol).

4   The Seven Day Plan For Women

Over the next seven pages you will find suggestions for eating including a breakdown of each meal's nutritional content. The three columns are designed so you may choose what appeals to you the most. If you do not see something you like, go to the next page. There are twenty-one different options for each meal over the seven days to choose from. Hopefully you will find foods that are appealing.

(a)   *Nutritional Content*

The nutritional breakdown is recorded as follows:

Calories / Fat / Protein / Total Carbs - Fiber - Net Carbs / Omega 6 - Omega 3 / Cholesterol

(b)   *Goals for the Seven Day Plan*

    (1) Try to keep your fiber intake at 10 grams per day or more
    (2) Drink your eight to twelve glasses of water per day to prevent constipation
    (3) Avoid carbohydrates early in the day to help maintain ketosis and lean body mass
    (4) You may add some fruit in the evening after supper (unless you are trying to lose weight)
    (5) Keep the ratio of omega-6 to omega-3 at 2:1 or better if possible
    (6) Experiment with new foods and new recipes (see recipes which follow)

Nutrition for Women

(Men, eat 50% more please)

Nutrition for Women (Men, eat 50% more please)

Nutritional Content
Calories / Fat / Protein / Total Carb - Fiber - Net Carbs / Omega 6 - Omega 3 / Cholesterol

Monday	Best	Better	Good
Breakfast	Smoked wild salmon (2 oz) (130/9/11/0/1-5/30) Eaten with a fork 1 Tbs. Cod liver oil (130/14/0/0/2-8/0) Green tea	2 poached eggs with (140/9/12/2-0-2/3-0/426) 2 strips organic turkey bacon (40/1/6/0/0-0/20) 1 Tbs. Cod liver oil (130/14/0/0/2-8/0) Decaf coffee	Hot organic Italian turkey sausage (one link-4 oz) (160/6/26/4-2-2/2-0/70) 1 Tbs. Cod liver oil (130/14/0/0/2-8/0) Coffee
Lunch	Salmon salad (½ cup) (288/21/21/3-2-1/4-3/62)	Tuna salad (½ cup) (205/12/22/0/3-2/37)	Chicken salad (½ cup) (206/18/31/5-2-3/4-0/70)
Snacks	30 almonds (1 oz) (180/16/7/7-4-3/4-0/0) Green tea	16 macadamia nuts (1 oz) (220/20/3/3-2-1/4-0/0) Decaf coffee	15 whole cashews (1 oz) (180/15/4/9-1-7/4-0/0) Coffee
Dinner	Filet Mignon (6 oz) (or other lean steak) with sautéed onion (338/27/48/6-2-4/3-0/130) Greens with garlic and olive oil (or other fat) (140/7/5/5-5-1/0-0/0)	Sautéed Flounder (8 oz) (320/13/38/6-2-4/1-2/100) Salad with 1 Tbs. Dressing (205/14/4/16-4-12/2-0/0)	Chicken stir fry (6 oz) (360/13/54/6-2-4/5-0/120) California style broccoli (175/11/9/12-6-6/3-0/0)

Monday	Best	Better	Good
Dessert Or snack	Strawberry Smoothie (140/9/6/13-7-6/2-3/0)	Strawberry Smoothie (140/9/6/13-7-6/2-3/0)	Strawberry Smoothie (140/9/6/13-7-6/2-3/0)
Calories Fat Protein CHO Fiber Net "carbs" O-6/O-3 Cholesterol	1285 calories 98 gm (882 cal- 68%) 88 gm (352 cal- 28%) 32 gm 20 gm 12 gm (48 calories- 4%) 14 gm/16 gm (1:1) 222 mg	1167 calories 79 gm (711 cal- 61%) 89 gm (356 cal- 30%) 42 gm 17 gm 25gm (100 calories-9%) 12 gm/12gm (1:1) 585 mg	1297 calories 77 gm (693 cal- 54%) 124 gm (496 cal- 38%) 47 gm 20 gm 27 gm (108 calories- 6%) 20 gm/ 8gm (2.5:1) 260 mg

CHO = carbohydrates

Please substitute from the Best, Better or Good columns; look to see what appeals to you most.

If you like coffee, drink it with and after your smoked salmon and tablespoon of cod liver oil.

If you like to drink a lot of coffee, drink brewed decaffeinated coffee (water extracted). It has 40% of the caffeine of regular coffee.

Nutrition for Women (Men, eat 50% more please)

Nutritional Content
Calories / Fat / Protein / Total Carbs - Fiber - Net Carbs / Omega 6 - Omega 3 / Cholesterol

Tuesday	Best	Better	Good
Breakfast	Leftover steak 2 oz (113/9/16/2-0-1/1-0/40) 1 Tbs. Cod liver oil (130/14/0/0/2-8/0) Green tea	Almond butter 2 Tbs. (180/16/7/7-4-2/4-0/0) 1 Tbs. Cod liver oil (130/14/0/0/2-8/0) Decaf coffee	2 soft-boiled eggs (140/9/12/2-0-2/3-0/426) 1 Tbs. Cod liver oil (130/14/0/0/2-8/0) Coffee
Lunch	Bristling Sardines in 2 layers 1 can (150/10/14/0/1-5/48)	4 oz sliced turkey rolled up w/ lettuce & spicy mustard (150/2/35/0/1-0/66)	4 oz sliced roast beef rolled up w/ lettuce & spicy mustard (230/9/34/0/2-0/90)
Snacks	30 almonds (1 oz) (180/16/7/7-4-2/4-0/0) Green tea	1 oz unsweetened chocolate (140/14/4/4-2-2/2-0) Decaf coffee	1 oz 70% chocolate (136/10/3/12-2-10/2-0/0) Coffee
Dinner	Salmon in dill sauce 6 oz (270/17/27/0/3-9/93) Salad with 2 Tbs. olive oil / rice vinegar dressing (170/14/2/6-2-4/2-0/0)	Broiled lamb 6 oz (344/16/46/0/2-0/155) Salad with 2 Tbs. olive oil / rice vinegar dressing (170/14/2/6-2-4/2-0/0)	Crustless crab and broccoli quiche (136/8/12/4-2-2/1-1/228) Salad with 2 Tbs. olive oil / rice vinegar dressing (170/14/2/6-2-4/2-0/0)

Tuesday	Best	Better	Good
Dessert Or bedtime snack	Blueberry Smoothie (157/9/6/18-8-10/2-3/0)	Blueberry Smoothie (157/9/6/18-8-10/2-3/0)	Blueberry Smoothie (157/9/6/18-8-10/2-3/0)
Calories Fat Protein CHO Fiber Net "carbs" O-6/O-3 Cholesterol	1038 calories 80 gm (720 calories- 69%) 66 gm (264 calories- 25%) 30 gm 16 gm 14 gm (56 calories- 5%) 13/21 (2:3) 181 mg	1004 calories 76 gm (684 cal- 68%) 94 gm (376 cal- 37%) 29 gm 16 gm 13 gm (52 calories- 5%) 13/8 (3:2) 221 mg	962 calories 64 gm (576 cal- 61%) 63 gm (252 cal- 27% 36 gm 14 gm 22 gm (88 calories- 10%) 12/9 (4:3) 744 mg

Balancing your fats: You must take an Omega-3 oil supplement (cod liver oil) to balance the ratio of omega-6 and omega-3 oils. Too much omega-6 oil appears to promote cancer growth.

If you are sick or over 70 years old, use the cod liver oil. The ALA in flax oil must be metabolized to EPA and DHA (the fish oils) which becomes less efficient with disease or older age.

Some people feel flax oil may increase prostate cancer in men; therefore it may be prudent to avoid the flax and take the cod liver oil instead.

Nutrition for Women (Men, eat 50% more please)

Nutritional Content
Calories / Fat / Protein / Total Carbs - Fiber - Net Carbs / Omega 6 - Omega 3 / Cholesterol

Wednesday	Best	Better	Good
Breakfast	2 eggs poached or coddled (140/9/12/2-0-2/3-0/426) with 2 oz of leftover salmon (90/6/9/0/2-6/31) 1 Tbs. Cod liver oil (130/14/0/0/2-8/0) Green tea	Fish sausage 4 oz (160/9/26/1-0-1/3-1/68) 1 Tbs. Cod liver oil (130/14/0/0/2-8/0) Decaf coffee	4 oz organic turkey Kielbasa (118/6/18/2-0-2/0-0/28) 1 Tbs. Cod liver oil (130/14/0/0/2-8/0) Coffee
Lunch	Kippers 1can (165/12/11/0/2-9/50)	Curried Tuna salad (½ cup) (205/13/22/0/3-2/37)	Leftover Quiche (1/4 of pie) (136/8/12/4-2-2/1-1/213)
Snacks	8 Brazil nuts (1 oz) (190/19/4/3-2-1/7-0/0) Green tea	14 pecan halves (1 oz) (200/20/3/4-2-2/9-0/0) Decaf coffee	14 walnut halves (1 oz) (180/17/4/3-2-1/11-0) Coffee
Dinner	Flounder fillet with shrimp (285/10/46/3-2-1/2-1/162) Sautéed Zucchini w/ garlic (83/7/2/4-2-2/1-0) Salad with 2 Tbs. olive oil & rice vinegar dressing (170/14/2/6-2-4/2-0/0)	Steak with onions 6 oz (338/27/48/6-2-4/3-0/150) Sautéed Zucchini (83/7/2/4-2-2/1-0/0)	Shrimp 4 oz with pesto (568/35/42/3-2-1/5-2/260) 8 asparagus stalks w/ lemon (60/0/6/12-4-8/0)

Wednesday	Best	Better	Good
Dessert Or bedtime snack	¼ cup blueberries (40/0/1/10-3-7/0)	¼ cup blueberries (40/0/1/10-3-7/0)	¼ cup blueberries (40/0/1/10-3-7/0)
Calories Fat Protein Carbohydrate Fiber Net "carbs" O-6/O-3 Cholesterol	1293 calories 91 gm (819 calories-63%) 87 gm (348 calories-27%) 28 gm 11 gm 17 gm (68 calories-5%) 21/32 669 mg	1259 calories 87 gm (783 cal - 62%) 102 gm (408 cal - 33%) 28 gm 11 gm 17 gm (68 cal - 5%) 20/10 257 mg	1136 calories 80 gm (720 cal-63%) 83 gm (332 cal-29%) 34 gm 13 gm 21 gm (84 cal-8%) 19/11 501 mg

Leave out dessert while you are losing weight.

The berries are much lower in carbohydrates and higher in fiber and antioxidants than other sweeter fruit from trees.

Nutrition for Women (Men, eat 50% more please)

Nutritional Content
Calories / Fat / Protein / Total Carbs - Fiber - Net Carbs / Omega 6 - Omega 3 / Cholesterol

Thursday	Best	Better	Good
Breakfast	2 eggs "over easy" with (140/9/12/2-0-2/3-0/426) 2 strips organic turkey bacon (40/1/6/0/0-0/20) 1 Tbs. Cod liver oil (130/14/0/0/2-8/0) Decaf coffee	Kippers 2 oz. in wine sauce (152/8/10/4-0-4/0-3/38) 1 Tbs. Cod liver oil (130/14/0/0/2-8/0) Decaf coffee	Kippers 2 oz. in cream sauce (152/8/10/4-0-4/0-3/38) 1 Tbs. Cod liver oil (130/14/0/0/2-8/0) Coffee
Lunch	Mixed green salad with hard-boiled egg and (103/5/8/8-2-6/1-0/213) 2 Tbs. Ranch dressing (193/20/0/2-0-2/2-0/21)	Leftover steak (2 oz) and zucchini (113/9/19/2-1-2/1-0/50)	Leftover shrimp pesto (2 oz) (184/12/14/1-0-0/2-1/84)
Snacks	14 pecan halves (1 oz) (200/20/3/4-2-2/9-0/0) Green tea	1 oz unsweetened chocolate (140/14/4/4-2-2/2-0/0) Decaf coffee	1 oz 70% chocolate (136/10/3/12-2-10/2-0/0) Coffee
Dinner	Flounder Creole (340/19/30/12-2-10/2-5/100) Salad with 2 Tbs. olive oil / rice vinegar dressing (170/14/2/6-2-4/2-0/0)	Shrimp and scallop stew (407/17/48/12-3-9/2-3/285) Salad with 2 Tbs. olive oil / rice vinegar dressing (170/14/2/6-2-4/2-0/0)	Italian pot roast (600/46/60/12-5-7/0-0/180) Salad with 2 Tbs. olive oil / rice vinegar dressing (170/14/2/6-2-4/2-0/0)

Thursday	Best	Better	Good
Dessert Or bedtime snack	Fresh Berries with Heavy Cream and Brandy (116/5/2/15-6-9/0/15)	Fresh Berries with Heavy Cream and Brandy (116/5/2/15-6-9/0/15)	Fresh Berries with Heavy Cream and Brandy (116/5/2/15-6-9/0/15)
Calories Fat gms Protein gms Carb gms Fiber gms Net carbs O-6/O-3 Cholesterol	1392 Calories 112 gm (1008 cal- 72%) 63 gm (252 cal- 18%) 47 gm 14 gm 33 gm (132 cal- 10%) 19/13 795 mg	1173 Calories 81 gm (729 cal-62%) 81 gm (324 cal-28%) 44 gm 14 gm 30 gm (120 cal-10%) 6/14 388 mg	1461 Calories 109 gm (981 cal-67%) 91 gm (364 cal-25%) 44 gm 15gm 29 gm (116 cal-8%) 6/12 317 mg

I still have some concerns about consuming too much saturated fat. We all have small vessel disease (little tiny strokes) when we do MRI scanning (a special type of picture of the brain) after age 50 years or so. Dr. Swank has shown that you can mimic these small strokes by injecting particles the size of saturated fat into animals.

If you are going to add alcohol to the diet, make sure you add in those carbohydrates. You will probably need to reduce some other carbohydrate, such as the berries or vegetables like zucchini or eggplant.

Nutrition for Women (Men, eat 50% more please)

Nutritional Content
Calories / Fat / Protein / Total Carbs - Fiber - Net Carbs / Omega 6 - Omega 3 / Cholesterol

Friday	Best	Better	Good
Breakfast	Smoked wild salmon (2 oz) (130/9/11/0/1-5/30) w/ sliced onion 1 Tbs. Cod liver oil (130/14/0/0/2-8/0) Green tea	Omelet w/ lox and sautéed onions (298/24/17/0/3-3/462) 1 Tbs. Cod liver oil (130/14/0/0/2-8/0) Decaf coffee	Organic ham and cheese omelet (376/30/28/0/3-0/487) 1 Tbs. Cod liver oil (130/14/0/0/2-8/0) Coffee
Lunch	Brisling sardines in 2 layers packed in olive oil, 1 can (156/10/48/0/1-5/48) 8 oz water	Tamari tuna salad (½ cup) (205/13/22/0/3-2/37) 8 oz water	Curried chicken salad (206/18/31/5-2-3/4-0/70) (½ cup) 8 oz water
Snacks	14 walnut halves (1 oz) (180/17/4/3-2-1/11-0/0) Green tea	8 Brazil nuts (1 oz) (190/19/4/3-2-1/7-0/0) Decaf coffee	14 pecan halves (1 oz) (200/20/3/4-2-2/9-0/0) Coffee
Dinner	Renaissance Greek Salad (anchovies optional) (600/50/18/20-6-14/2-0/44)	Irish chicken dinner (378/18/41/11-6-5/4-0/120)	Irish lamb soup (470/26/44/9-5-4/2-0/135)
Dessert Or bedtime snack	8 fresh strawberries (25/0/1/5-2-3/0/0)	8 fresh strawberries (25/0/1/5-2-3/0/0)	8 fresh strawberries (25/0/1/5-2-3/0/0)

Friday	Best	Better	Good
Calories	1300 calories	1168 calories	1340 calories
Fat gms	100 gm (900 cal-69%)	88 gm 792 cal-68%)	96 gm (864 calories-65%)
Protein gms	82 gm (328 cal-25%)	85 gm (340 cal-29%)	107 gm (428 cal-32%)
Carb gms	28 gm	19 gm	23 gm
Fiber gms	10 gm	10 gm	11 gm
Net carbs	18 gm (72 calories-6%)	9 gm (36 calories-3%)	12 gm (48 calories-3%)
O-6/O-3	17/18	19/13	18/8
Cholesterol	122 mg	619 mg	692 mg

Women will need to eat 1200 to 1300 calories per day to lose weight consistently. Men can eat 1800 to 2000 and often still lose weight.

If you are exercising, you can certainly increase your calories. I would not suggest just increasing your carbohydrates, but try to maintain these ratios of fat/carbohydrate/protein.

Eat more fruit if you would like to gain a little weight. The fruit trees bear fruit in the fall to fatten us up for the long cold winter. But now the grocery stores are open year-round and our houses have heat (although our children claim I never actually turn it on).

Nutrition for Women (Men, eat 50% more please)

Nutritional Content
Calories / Fat / Protein / Total Carbs - Fiber - Net Carbs / Omega 6 - Omega 3 / Cholesterol

Saturday	Best	Better	Good
Breakfast	The Japanese Breakfast (400/21/18/8-2-6/5-7/243) Green tea	Goat Cheese omelet (336/28/23/0/3-0/469) 1 Tbs. Cod liver oil (130/14/0/0/2-8/0) Decaf coffee	Oat waffles (339/23/10/22-2-20/0/160) w/ strawberries & cream 78/6/1/11-4-7/0-0/21) 1 Tbs. Cod liver oil (130/14/0/0/2-8/0) Coffee
Lunch	The Japanese Lunch (130/9/11/0-0-0/1-5/30) 8 oz water	Leftover Irish chicken dinner (1/2 serving) (189/9/20/5-3-2/2-0/60)	Leftover Irish lamb soup (1/2 serving) (300/20/22/5-2-3/1-0/68)
Snacks	Mixed nuts 2 oz 360/32/14/14-8-6/8-2/0) Green tea	1 oz unsweetened chocolate (140/14/4/4-2-2/2-0/0) Decaf coffee	1 oz 70% chocolate (136/10/3/12-2-10/2-0/0) Coffee
Dinner	The Japanese Dinner (430/30/29/8-2-6/6-12/60) Glass of dry white wine (85/0/0/3-0-3/0-0/0)	Baked chicken w/ basil (319/14/44/8-2-6/5-0/226) Salad with 2 Tbs. olive oil / rice vinegar dressing (170/14/2/6-2-4/2-0/0)	Mexican chicken salad (296/17/25/13-5-8/1-0/80) Black-eyed peas with garlic and kale (226/14/12/22-9-13/2-0/0)

Saturday	Best	Better	Good
Dessert Or bedtime snack	1 Kiwi, sliced (46/0/1/11-3-8/0/0)	½ cup blueberries fresh or frozen (42/0/1/10-3-7/0/0)	½ cup raspberries fresh or frozen 1 Tbs. heavy cream (88/6/1/9-4-5/0/21)
Calories Fat gms Protein gms Carb gms Fiber gms Net carbs O-6/O-3 Cholesterol	1220 calories 92 gm (828 calories-68%) 72 gm (288 calories-24%) 41 gm 15 gm 26 gm (104 calories-9%) 13/25 349 mg	1297 calories 93 gm (837 cal-65%) 94 gm (376 cal-29%) 33 gm 12 gm 21 gm (84 calories-6%) 16/8 755 mg	1514 calories 110 gm (990 cal-65%) 76 gm (304 cal-20%) 83 gm 28 gm 55 gm (220 calories-15%) 8/8 350 mg

The waffles are on the edge of acceptable, but I admit I do make them for the kids. Instead of syrup they use whipped cream (out of a can!). But life is full of compromises.

But if you go to one of those $15 buffet brunches with all of the wonderful fish and Eggs Benedict, don't eat the darn waffles. The fish and other great foods are worth much more to your body (and their pocketbook).

I hate to admit it but I always think the less informed are choosing the waffles and pastries instead of the salmon, mackerel, herring and fancy breakfast meats.

Nutrition for Women (Men, eat 50% more please)

Nutritional Content

Calories / Fat / Protein / Total Carbs - Fiber - Net Carbs / Omega 6 - Omega 3 / Cholesterol

Sunday	Best	Better	Good
Breakfast	Low Carb Waffles with Blueberries and cream (258/11/22/6-3-2/5-1/104) 1 Tbs. Cod liver oil (130/14/0/0/2-8/0) Green tea	2 eggs poached (140/9/12/2-0-2/3-0/426) w/ 2 Tbs. salsa 1 Tbs. Cod liver oil (130/14/0/0/2-8/0) Decaf coffee	Western omelet (262/21/14/4-1-3/2-1/556) 1 Tbs. Cod liver oil (130/14/0/0/2-8/0) Coffee
Lunch	Salmon cakes (260/22/18/3-2-1/6-5/50) Steamed greens of choice (140/7/5/5-5-1/0-0/0)	Crab cakes (190/11/9/3-2-1/0-2/50) Steamed greens of choice (140/7/5/5-5-1/0-0/0)	Shrimp salad (220/11/24/4-2-2/5-1/173)
Snacks	16 macadamia nuts (1 oz) (220/20/3/3-2-1/4-0/0) Green tea	14 walnut halves (1 oz) (180/17/4/3-2-1/11-0/0) Decaf coffee	15 whole cashews (1 oz) (180/15/4/9-1-7/4-0/0) Coffee
Dinner	Curried Chicken Salad with Grapes and Celery (287/14/25/14-2-12/4-1/85) Salad with 2 Tbs. olive oil & rice vinegar dressing (170/14/2/6-2-4/2-0/0)	Herbed Lamb Chops w/ asparagus (506/30/46/13-5-8/0-0/155) Salad with 2 Tbs. olive oil / rice vinegar dressing (170/14/2/6-2-4/2-0/0)	Beef and mushroom stew (293/17/18/10-2-7/0-0/125) Salad with 2 Tbs. olive oil / rice vinegar dressing (170/14/2/6-2-4/2-0/0)

Sunday	Best	Better	Good
Dessert Or bedtime snack	8 fresh strawberries (25/0/1/5-2-3/0/0)	½ cup blueberries fresh or frozen (42/0/1/10-3-7/0/0)	½ cup mixed berries fresh or frozen 1 Tbs. heavy cream (88/6/1/9-4-5/0/21)
Calories Fat gms Protein gms Carb gms Fiber gms Net carbs O-6/O-3 Cholesterol	1129 calories 81 gm (729 calories-65%) 76 gm (304 calories-26%) 42 gm 18 gm 24 gm (96 calories-9%) 23/15 239 gm	1153 calories 85 gm (765 cal-66%) 74 gm (296 cal-26%) 42 gm 19 gm 23 gm (92 calories-8%) 16/10 631 gm	1254 calories 98 gm (882 calories-%) 63 gm (252 calories-%) 42 gm 12 gm 30 gm (120 calories-%) 20/10 875 gm

Delicious and Healthy

Coming up!

Recipes for Monday

Breakfast

Smoked salmon Serves 1 (130/9/11/0/1-5/16)
2 oz of wild smoked salmon (not farm-raised)

You will be paying a high price ($10-$30/lb.) but it is worth it. The farming of salmon is damaging our coastal environments. The salmon are fed fish food (similar to dog food?) with food dyes and antibiotics to prevent infections in the dense populations in the pens. We owe it to the environment and ourselves to choose appropriately.

Two poached eggs Serves 1 (140/9/12/2-0-2/3-0/426) **with 2 strips organic turkey bacon** (40/1/6/0/0-0/20)

2 eggs
A sliver of butter or dash of olive oil
2 strips of turkey bacon
Salt and pepper to taste

2 dashes of beef bouillon powder (no MSG)
Dash of soy sauce or hot sauce is optional

Put a little water into a small pot and place egg poacher tray in pot and turn heat on high. Drop the butter or olive oil in poacher and wait for butter to melt. Carefully break the egg into the poacher. Bring to boil, cover and reduce heat and cook for 4 minutes (runny egg) to 6 minutes (medium egg). Meanwhile, cook the bacon in a separate pan. Or you could grab 2 ounces of sausage from the refrigerator (approximately 2 inches of a large sausage link). Slide the eggs into a warm bowl and enjoy. A dash of soy, hot sauce or the beef bouillon powder is a nice variation.

Hot organic Italian turkey sausage (160/6/26/4-2-2/2-0/70)
4 oz (one link) of organic Italian turkey sausage
1 Tsp. butter or olive oil

On Sunday evening while making dinner, cook 3-4 links (one package) of organic Turkey sausage. Heat the sausage and butter/oil in a heavy skillet at medium-high heat. Cook until the sausage is brown, turning frequently (8-10 minutes). Cover skillet and let "coast" for another10-15 minutes. Remove from heat, cut into bite-size pieces and place in a container in the refrigerator to enjoy for breakfasts or snacks during the week.

Lunch

Salmon salad Serves 2 with ½ cup each (288/21/21/3-2-1/4-3/60)

7.5 oz can of salmon-boneless	Salt and pepper to taste
2 Tbs. Grape seed oil mayonnaise	Optional: 1 Tbs. Chopped onion
2 celery stalks, finely chopped	

Mix all ingredients together. May serve with mixed green salad.

Helen of Troy salad of tuna Serves 1 (228/11/31/3-2-1/3-1/37)

6 oz can of solid white tuna, drained	1 celery stalk, finely chopped
1 Tbs. grape seed oil mayonnaise	Salt and pepper to taste
½ Tsp. Fresh dill or ¼ Tsp. dried dill	Optional: 1 Tbs. Chopped onion

Mix all ingredients together. May serve with mixed green salad.

Call me Ishmael's chicken/turkey salad (Serves 2 with ½ cup each) (206/18/31/5-2-3/4-0/80)

½ lb. boiled chicken or turkey breast	1 Tsp. lemon juice
1 Tbs. grape seed oil mayonnaise	2 celery stalks- finely chopped
1 Tbs. organic heavy cream	Salt and pepper to taste
½ Tbs. seasoned rice vinegar	Optional: 1 Tbs. Chopped onion

Mix all ingredients together. May serve with mixed green salad.

Snacks

Almonds (1 oz is 30 unroasted nuts) (180/16/7/7-4-3/4-0/0)

Almonds are high in fiber and monounsaturated fat. One to two ounces of almonds for snacking is appropriate if you are trying to lose weight. Three to five ounces is acceptable if you are maintaining your weight.

Macadamia nuts (1 oz is 16 nuts) (220/20/3/3-2-1/4-0/0)

Macadamia nuts are the lowest nuts in carbohydrate content, although they do not have as much fiber as almonds. But I love them (usually roasted and salted unfortunately). But avoid the salt if your ankles swell.

Cashews (1 oz is 15 whole nuts or 30 half nuts) (180/15/4/9-2-7/4-0/0)

Cashews are much higher in carbohydrates and lower in monounsaturated fat. But you may add them to your mixed nuts for some variety and richness of flavor. Do not overdo these if you are trying to lose weight.

Dinner

Filet mignon (or other lean steak) with sautéed onions (1 dinner / 1 breakfast) (338/27/48/6-2-4/3-0/130)

8 oz filet mignon	1 Tbs. organic butter
1 medium onion, sliced	Salt and pepper to taste
½ pound mushrooms, sliced	

Heat heavy skillet until hot. Add butter, mushrooms and onion and sauté until limp (1-2 minutes). Add filet and sear the first side until brown (1-2 minutes). Turn and sear second side as the first. Cover and turn off heat. Let sit for 3-5 minutes. The steak will be rare or medium rare, depending on the thickness. You may cook longer if you desire.

Sautéed flounder Serves 2 (320/13/38/6-2-4/1-2/100)

1 lb. Flounder fillet	¼ Tsp. red pepper
1 medium onion, sliced	Salt to taste
2 Tbs. Fresh parsley, chopped finely	Dash of soy sauce
1 Tbs. Organic butter or olive oil	

Heat heavy skillet until hot. Add butter and onion, reduce heat and sauté until limp (1-2 minutes). Add fillet and cook the first side until fish is no longer translucent (3-4 minutes). Turn and cook second side as the first. Cover and turn off heat. Let sit for 3-5 minutes. The fish will be easy to pull apart with a fork when done.

Calories / Fat / Protein / Total Carbs-Fiber-Net Carbs / Omega 6-Omega 3 / Cholesterol

Chicken stir-fry Serves 2 (360/13/54/6-2-4/5-0/120)

12 oz Chicken breast cut into 1/2-inch-wide strips	½ Tsp. salt
1 Tbs. olive oil	½ Tsp. dried thyme
1 medium onion, sliced	1/8 Tsp. ground red pepper
1 clove garlic, minced	2 Tbs. chopped fresh parsley
1 Tsp. curry powder	

Add olive oil and chicken to skillet. Stir-fry over medium-high heat for 3 minutes or until lightly browned. Add onion and garlic; stir-fry 3 minutes or until tender. Add curry powder and next 4 ingredients; stir well. Reduce heat. Simmer for 10-15 minutes or until tender. Spoon into bowls and sprinkle with parsley.

Vegetables

Greens with garlic and olive oil or other fat Serves 2 (140/7/5/5-5-1/0-0/0)

1 Tbs. olive oil or organic butter	1 Tbs. water
16-oz package frozen Kale (or 3 cups fresh, chopped)	Freshly ground pepper to taste
	1 large cloves garlic, crushed in press

   (Or may try collards, turnip or mustard greens)

Heat the water, kale (or other greens) and garlic in a large skillet over medium-high heat stirring until they are wilted. Simmer until the greens are tender, about 5 minutes, stirring occasionally; season to taste with salt and pepper. Remove from heat, add olive oil and stir to mix. Serve immediately.

California style broccoli with grape seed oil mayonnaise Serves 2 (175/11/9/12-6-6/3-0/0)

1 lb. Broccoli (12 spears)
2 Tbs. Grape seed oil mayonnaise

Steam broccoli for 3-5 minutes. Serve immediately with topping of mayonnaise.

Salad Serves 4 (65/0/4/14-4-10/0-0/0)

12 oz red leaf lettuce or mixed greens (8 cups)
1 medium cucumber, sliced

Nobel Prize winning vinaigrette Serves 2 (140/14/0/2-0-2/2-0/0)

2 Tbs. olive oil	½ dried tarragon
2 Tbs. Rice vinegar	½ Tsp. Dried mustard
2 fresh basil leaves; chopped or 1 Tsp. dried basil	¼ Tsp. Sea salt
	Ground pepper to taste

Salad with dressing (205/14/4/16-4-12/2-0) No nitrites or other preservatives in the turkey or roast beef

Dessert

Strawberry smoothie Serves 2 (140/9/6/13-7-6/2-3/0)

1 cup frozen strawberries	½ Tsp. vanilla
15 almonds	(1 pack of Stevia)
1 cup filtered water	

Place the nuts in the blender and blend until chopped into fine pieces. Add the water and blend on high, adding the strawberries one at a time. Blend for 2-3 minutes or until thick. Pour immediately into two bowls and enjoy.

Leftover filet mignon 2 oz (113/9/16/2-0-1/1-0/44)

I usually eat the filet cold out of the refrigerator, followed by the supplements. Then I swallow a tablespoon of cod liver oil. I drink decaffeinated coffee with a touch of heavy cream on the way to work.

Almond butter 2 Tbs. (180/16/7/7-4-2/4-0/0)

I scoop the almond butter into a bowl and then eat it with a spoon. Then I swallow a tablespoon of cod liver oil. I drink decaffeinated coffee with a touch of heavy cream on the way to work (again).

Soft-boiled egg with leftover sausage (150/10/19/1-0-1/0-1/248)

1 egg	Salt and pepper to taste
2 pieces of leftover sausage (2 oz)	1 Tsp. salsa (optional)

Place egg and the sausage in a pot of cold water and place on high heat. Bring to boil, reduce heat to low and cover. Let cook for 3-4 minutes. Then remove sausage to a plate. Place egg under cold water to cool. Shell egg, salt and pepper to taste.

Lunch

Bristling sardines in 2 layers (serves 1) (150/10/14/0/1-5/48)

1 can, eaten with a fork. The best sardines are the "Bristling Sardines in two layers" because they are small. This means you cannot appreciate the bones or other components more obvious in the larger sardines. You may choose the lightly smoked ones, but (unfortunately) the smoke may not be that good for you (but isn't life full of compromises? Yes!).

Sliced turkey rolled up with lettuce and spicy mustard (150/2/35/0/1-0/66)

4 oz sliced turkey. Turkey tends to be one of the cleanest of meats. Turkeys will die if you raise them in unhealthy environments, as opposed to chickens which can be treated atrociously and still survive only to end up on your table full of hormones and antibiotics. But if you can afford to buy organic with no nitrites or other preservatives, all the better!

Sliced roast beef rolled up with lettuce and spicy mustard (230/9/34/0/2-0/90)

4 oz of sliced organic roast beef without preservatives rolled up with lettuce and spicy mustard and held together with a toothpick.

Snack

Chocolate (Ah, the sex surrogate)

Unsweetened chocolate is just a drug (but you love it). The 70% chocolate is a definite compromise, but perhaps one worth making for those of you who do not like the Baker's unsweetened. It does take a little getting used to, but as with spinach or broccoli or kale or collard greens, the training of the palate is important. Better living through chemistry. Avoid this if your allergies or asthma seems to be worse while eating this and better while not eating this (this is my experience, unfortunately- I guess I'll just have to have more sex?).

Dinner

Salmon fillets with mustard and mayo glaze (2 servings & 2 lunches) (492/37/36/2-0-2/17-9/93)
> Calories 337, Fat 25, Mono 10, Poly 6/4, Sat 5, Carbohydrate 10, Sugar 9, Fiber 1, Protein 18

1 lb. Salmon fillet, cut into 4 equal pieces	1 Tbs. lemon juice
4 Tbs. Grape seed oil mayonnaise	4 or 5 cloves garlic, pressed
2 Tbs. spicy mustard	

Place salmon in a shallow baking dish. Blend remaining ingredients together in a bowl and spread evenly over top of salmon fillets. Place under heated broiler for 5 minutes. Turn off oven keeping oven door closed and let "coast" for an additional 5-10 minutes or until the salmon is just opaque in the center. Transfer to a serving platter and serve immediately.

Broiled lamb kebobs Serves 4 (350/19/36/8-3-5/2-0/ 108)

1 lb. Boneless lamb loin	Salt and freshly ground pepper to taste
2 Tbs. olive oil	8 small onions, peeled
2 Tbs. Lemon juice	1 small red pepper
1 Tsp. Oregano	1 small yellow or green pepper

Cut the lamb into 1-inch cubes. Place the cubes in a glass dish and sprinkle with lemon juice, oregano, and salt and pepper to taste. Peel the onions and sauté the whole onions in olive oil 10 to 15 minutes or until almost tender. Seed the peppers and cut them into 1 1/2-inch pieces.

Thread the lamb alternating with vegetables onto flat-bladed metal skewers. Preheat the broiler. Place the skewers on a broiling pan and cook about 5 inches from the heat, turning every 3 to 4 minutes, for 12 minutes or until meat is brown outside but still pink inside.

Crustless crab and broccoli quiche Serves 6 (136/8/12/4-2-2/1-1/245)

1 Tbs. olive oil	1 (6-ounce) can lump crabmeat, drained
1 cup chopped fresh broccoli	½ cup almond milk
½ cup finely chopped sweet red pepper	½ Tsp. salt
¼ cup finely chopped onion	¼ Tsp. dry mustard
¼ cup water	¼ Tsp. ground red pepper
4 large eggs, lightly beaten	

Combine broccoli, sweet red pepper, onion, and olive oil in a medium saucepan. Cover and cook over medium heat 3 to 5 minutes or until vegetables are crisp-tender. Combine vegetable mixture, beaten eggs and next 6 ingredients in a large bowl, stirring well. Pour mixture into a 9-inch quiche dish coated with cooking spray. Bake at 350° for 35 to 40 minutes or until set. Let stand 10 minutes before slicing into 6 wedges.

Dessert

Blueberry smoothie Serves 2 (157/9/6/18-8-10/2-3/0)

1 cup frozen blueberries	½ Tsp. vanilla
15 almonds	(1 pack of Stevia)
1 cup filtered water	

Place nuts in blender and blend until chopped into fine pieces. Add the water and blend on high while adding the blueberries. Blend for 2-3 minutes or until thick. Pour immediately into two bowls and enjoy.

Two coddled eggs with salmon Serves 2 (140/9/12/2-0-2/3-0/426) & (90/6/9/0/2-6/)

2 eggs	Salt and pepper to taste
1 Tsp. butter	2 oz. of leftover salmon
2 Egg Coddlers	

Fill a pot of water enough to immerse the coddlers to just below their lids (about 2/3 the way up the coddler) and heat to boiling. Place ½ Tsp. of butter in each coddler, cover and place in boiling water for 1 minute to melt the butter. Remove the coddlers and carefully break 1 egg into each coddler, cover and return to boiling water for 4 minutes. Remove from water and serve immediately. May be eaten directly from the coddler.

Organic Italian turkey sausage (serves 1) (160/6/26/4-2-2/2-0/70)

Buy the package of 3 or 4 sausages and cook them up on Sunday. Put them in a bowl with plastic wrap in the refrigerator to have throughout the week. One sausage is a 4 oz serving.

Organic turkey kielbasa (serves 1) (118/6/18/2-0-2/0-0/28)

The nice thing about this is the Kielbasa is already fully cooked, so you can snack on it whenever you want. You may heat it or eat it cold. Each 1 inch of sausage is approximately 1 oz, so 3-4 inches is a serving (4 oz).

Lunch

Kippers Serves 1 (165/12/11/0/2-9)
Kippered herring 3.75 oz. can

If you like smoked oysters, you will probably like kippers. They are not like sardines at all. I don't even like sardines but I eat them because they are good for you. Kippers have no bones (and therefore not rich in calcium) and have the consistency of tuna.

Calories / Fat / Protein / Total Carbs-Fiber-Net Carbs / Omega 6-Omega 3 / Cholesterol

Curried tuna salad Serves 1 (228/11/31/3-2-1/3-1/37)

6 oz can of solid white tuna, drained   ½ Tsp. curry powder

1 Tbs. Grape seed oil mayonnaise   Salt and pepper to taste

1 celery stalk, finely chopped

Mix all ingredients together. May serve with mixed green salad.

Snacks

Brazil nuts (1 oz is 8 nuts) (190/19/4/3-2-1/7-0/0)

Brazil nuts are rich in selenium, which appears to reduce cancer of the colon, prostate and lung. They are very low in carbohydrates but higher in omega-6 oils. Be sure to take the cod liver oil or eat your sardines or kippers if you are going to eat these.

Pecans (1 oz is 14 pecan halves) (200/20/3/4-2-2/9-0/0)

Pecans are also high in omega-6 oils, but their high fat content make them taste very rich.

Walnuts (1 oz is 14 walnut halves) (180/17/4/3-2-1/??/0)

Walnuts have the highest omega-3 content of all of the tree nuts and are very low in carbohydrates.

Dinner

Flounder fillet with shrimp Serves 2 (285/10/46/3-2-1/2-1/162)

2 onion slices	4 flounder fillets (4 ounces each)
1 Tsp. lemon juice	Salt and freshly ground black pepper
2 parsley sprigs	¼ pound mushrooms, sliced
1 bay leaf	1 cup water
¼ Tsp. ground thyme	1 Tbs. olive oil
12 small shrimp, shelled and deveined (4 oz)	

Preheat oven to 325° F. Sauté the mushrooms onion slices in the olive oil. Add the lemon juice, parsley, bay leaf, thyme, and water. Bring mixture to a boil. Add the shrimp, and cook them for three to five minutes.

Place the flounder fillets in a double layer in a two-inch-deep baking dish, seasoning between the layers with salt and pepper. Pour the sauce over the fish, cover and bake for fifteen to twenty minutes or until the fish flakes easily when tested with a fork. Garnish with shrimp and place under the broiler until lightly browned and bubbly hot.

Steak with onions Serves 2 (338/27/48/6-2-4/3-0/150)

2-one inch thick steaks 6 oz. each	1 Tbs. Butter or olive oil
1 small onion	Salt and pepper to taste

Slice onion and sauté in butter or oil in a heavy pan. Reserve onion, heat pan to hot and sear steak on each side (2-3 minutes). Return onions to pan and cover while turning off the heat. The heavy pan will continue to slowly cook the steak for the next 10-15 minutes. The result should be medium rare. If you prefer your steak more done, extend the initial cooking time to 4-5 minutes.

Shrimp with pesto Serves 2 (568/35/42/3-2-1/5-2/260)

12 oz fresh or frozen shrimp	¼ cup olive oil
1 cup fresh basil	1 Tbs. grated Parmesan cheese
1 large garlic clove, pressed	

Add basil, garlic and olive oil to blender and blend on medium-high until basil is completely chopped and mixed with olive oil. Add Parmesan cheese and blend until mix. Let set while cooking shrimp.

Boil water in medium pot, add shrimp and cook for 3-4 minutes for fresh shrimp or 4-6 minutes for frozen shrimp. Drain shrimp and place in bowl. Pour pesto sauce over the shrimp, stir and serve immediately or may keep in refrigerator to serve later.

Calories / Fat / Protein / Total Carbs-Fiber-Net Carbs / Omega 6-Omega 3 / Cholesterol

Vegetables

Sautéed zucchini with garlic (83/7/2/4-2-2/1-0/0)

2 small or one large zucchini, sliced 1/4 inch thick

1 Tbs. olive oil

1 clove garlic, crushed in a press

1/4 Tsp. red and black pepper

Add olive oil to skillet; cook the zucchini and onion over medium heat. Add the remaining ingredients and cook on low heat for 3 minutes or until the zucchini has reached a desired tenderness.

Sautéed zucchini with onion (83/7/2/4-2-2/1-0)

2 small or one large zucchini, sliced 1/4 inch thick

1 medium onion, sliced into 1/4 inch wedges

1 Tbs. olive oil

2 dashes of red and black pepper

Add olive oil to skillet; cook the zucchini and onion over medium heat. Add the remaining ingredients and cook on low heat for 3 minutes or until the zucchini has reached a desired tenderness.

Asparagus with lemon (60/0/6/12-4-8/0)

14 spears of asparagus

1 Tsp. butter

1 Tbs. water

1 Tbs. lemon juice

Place all ingredients in skillet and heat to steaming. Cover and simmer on low for 4-6 minutes. Remove from heat and serve immediately on a warm plate.

Dessert

Blueberry smoothie Serves 2 (157/9/6/18-8-10/2-3/0)

1 cup frozen blueberries

15 almonds

1 cup filtered water

½ Tsp. vanilla

(1 pack of Stevia)

Place nuts in blender and blend until chopped into fine pieces. Add the water and blend on high, adding the blueberries slowly. Blend for 2-3 minutes or until thick. Pour immediately into two bowls and enjoy.

Recipes for Thursday

Breakfast

Two eggs over-easy (140/9/12/2-0-2/3-0/426) **with organic turkey bacon**
(40/1/6/0/0-0/70) Serves 1

2 eggs   1 Tbs. Butter or olive oil
2 slices of organic turkey bacon

     First heat the oil/butter and turkey bacon in a heavy skillet. Cook bacon until done to your liking (crisp or otherwise). Scrape pan (leaving the "stuff" along the sides) and add eggs to skillet on medium-low heat. You may need to add a little more oil/butter before adding eggs. When whites are solidified, flip the eggs (cover for "sunny side up" eggs). Turn off heat to prevent overcooking.

Kippers in wine sauce (rinsed) (in bottles found in the refrigerated section of the grocery store) (152/8/10/4-0-4/0-3/38)
3 oz of kippers, rinsed in water (approximately 1/3 cup of kippers)

     Enjoy with a knife and fork.

Kippers in cream sauce (rinsed) (in bottles found in the refrigerated section of the grocery store) (152/8/10/4-0-4/0-3/38)
3 oz of kippers, rinsed in water (approximately 1/3 cup of kippers)

     Enjoy with a knife and fork.

Lunch

Mixed green salad with hard-boiled egg Serves 2 (103/5/8/8-2-6/1-0/213)
4 cups (1/2 lb.) mixed greens or lettuce   1 hard boiled egg, sliced
½ cucumber, sliced thinly

     Mix all ingredients and serve in large shallow bowls. Put anchovies as desired on salads. Place decanters of olive oil and rice vinegar on the table for individuals to serve themselves as needed. Add Ranch dressing or olive oil and vinegar.

Ranch dressing Serves 2 193/20/0/2-0-2/2-0/21)

1 Tbs. olive oil	Dash of onion powder
1 Tbs. organic heavy cream	Salt and pepper to taste
1 Tbs. Rice vinegar	Dash of garlic powder (optional, but good!)
1 Tsp. Lemon juice	

Mix ingredients well and pour on salad. (I agree that adding the organic heavy cream is a compromise, but use the rest in your decaffeinated coffee?)

Leftover steak with zucchini Serves 1 (113/9/19/2-1-2/1-0/50)

Save 2 oz of steak (that is ½ the size of your palm) from the dinner the night before for your lunch today.

Leftover shrimp with pesto Serves 1 (184/12/14/1-0-0/2-1/84)

Save 1/3 cup of the Shrimp dish from dinner the night before to eat for your lunch today.

Dinner

Flounder Creole Serves 2 (340/19/30/12-2-10/2-5/100)

Flounder fillets 1 lb.	1 Tbs. Worcestershire sauce
2 Tbs. olive oil	1 Tbs. rice vinegar
½ red onion, chopped	3/4 Tsp. dried basil
2 cloves garlic, crushed	1/4 Tsp. salt
7 oz can of whole tomatoes, undrained and chopped	Pinch ground red pepper

Heat oil in large skillet or wok over medium heat. Add onion and garlic and sauté until tender. Add tomato and remaining ingredients except fish. Bring to a boil. Add fillets, spooning tomato mixture over fish. Reduce heat, cover and simmer 12 minutes.

Shrimp, crab and scallop stew (Serves 2 plus two 1/3 cup lunch servings) (407/17/48/13-3-10/2-3/285)

2 Tbs. olive oil

½ cup chopped onion

1 clove garlic, minced

7 oz can of whole tomatoes, undrained and chopped

¼ cup chopped fresh oregano

2 Tbs. chopped fresh parsley

1 Tsp. low-sodium Worcestershire sauce

1/8 Tsp. red pepper

½ pound bay scallops (fresh or frozen)

½ pound medium-size shrimp, peeled and de-veined (fresh or frozen)

2 oz. can of white crab meat

Add the olive oil to the pot; place over medium-high heat until hot. Add chopped onion, sweet red pepper, add minced garlic; sauté until vegetables are tender. Add tomato, stirring well to combine. Add oregano and next 3 ingredients; stir well. Bring vegetable mixture to a boil over medium heat; cover, reduce heat, and simmer 20 minutes. Add scallops and shrimp to vegetable mixture; bring to a boil. Reduce heat, and simmer 7 to 8 minutes or until scallops and shrimp are done.

Italian pot roast (2 dinner servings and a lunch) (600/46/60/12-5-7/0-0/180)

1 lb. organic beef roast cut into 2-inch cubes

¼ lb. hot organic Italian sausage

1 medium onion, chopped

3 garlic cloves, pressed

2 carrots cut into 1-inch pieces

4 celery stalks, cut into 1-inch pieces

1 red pepper, chopped

12 mushrooms, sliced

2 Tbs. fresh chopped parsley

½ Tsp. thyme

½ Tsp. oregano

1 Tsp. basil

½ Tsp. cayenne pepper

1/8-Tsp. fennel seeds

2 Tbs. olive oil

1 Tbs. organic butter

2 Tbs. organic heavy cream

1 cup water

Heat olive oil and butter in large pot. Sauté beef and sausage for 5 minutes or until browned. Add onion and garlic and sauté for additional 5 minutes. Add remaining ingredients, bring to boil, cover and reduce heat and simmer for 1-1/2 to 2 hours or until beef is tender. Serve in bowls.

Dessert

Fresh berries with heavy cream and brandy Serves 2 (116/5/2/15-6-9/0/15)

½ cup fresh blueberries

½ cup fresh raspberries

1 cup fresh strawberries, halved

2 Tbs. organic heavy cream

2 Tsp. Brandy

Mix berries and distribute evenly into two shallow bowls. Pour 1 Tbs. of cream followed by 1 Tsp. Brandy on fruit.

Recipes for Friday

Breakfast

Omelet w/ lox and sautéed onions Serves 1 (298/24/17/0/3-3/462)

2 eggs
1 Tbs. organic heavy cream
1 Tbs. chopped onion

1 oz. lox or nova salmon cut into small
pieces
1 Tsp. olive oil or butter
Salt and pepper to taste

Beat eggs and cream until mixed. Put olive oil or butter in shallow pan over medium heat. Sauté onion and reserve. Pour egg mixture into pan and swish pan to spread the egg mixture over the pan. Reduce heat to low and add the onion and lox over half of the egg mixture. Flip the other half over the lox and onions. Cook 2-3 more minutes, flipping omelet once.

Organic ham and cheese omelet Serves 1 (376/30/28/0/3-0/487)

2 eggs
1 Tbs. heavy cream
1 oz. goat cheese, crumbled

1 oz. organic ham or turkey, chopped
1 Tbs. butter
Salt and pepper to taste

Beat eggs and cream until mixed. Put olive oil or butter in shallow pan over medium heat. Pour egg mixture into pan and swish pan to spread the egg mixture over the pan. Reduce heat to low and add the cheese and ham over half of the egg mixture. Flip the other half over the cheese and ham. Cook 2-3 more minutes, flipping omelet once.

Lunch

Brisling sardines in 2 layers packed in olive oil 1 can (156/10/48/0/1-5/48)

Tamari tuna salad Serves 1 (228/11/31/3-2-1/3-1)

6 oz can of solid white tuna, drained
1 Tbs. Grape seed oil mayonnaise
1 celery stalk, finely chopped

½ Tsp. Tamari sauce
Salt and pepper to taste

Mix all ingredients together. May serve with mixed green salad.

Calories / Fat / Protein / Total Carbs-Fiber-Net Carbs / Omega 6-Omega 3 / Cholesterol

Curried chicken salad Serves 2 (206/18/31/5-2-3/4-0)

½ lb. boiled chicken or turkey breast	2 celery stalks- finely chopped
1 Tbs. Grape seed oil mayonnaise	1 Tsp. Curry powder
½ Tbs. Seasoned rice vinegar	Salt and pepper to taste
1 Tsp. lemon juice	Optional: 1 Tbs. Chopped onion

Mix all ingredients together. May serve with mixed green salad.

Dinner

Renaissance Greek salad (Serves 2 adults) (600/50/18/20-6-14/2-0/44)

4 cups (6 oz) mixed greens or lettuce	4 oz. Feta (goat) cheese, crumbled
12 mushrooms, quartered	¼ cup olive oil
1 large tomato, chopped	1 Tbs. lemon juice
1 green pepper, chopped	1 Tbs. rice vinegar
¼ Bermuda onion, thinly sliced	½ Tsp. oregano leaves
10 Black olives (pitted or non-pitted)	Salt and pepper to taste
½ cucumber, sliced thinly	Optional: 1 small can of anchovies

Mix salad ingredients and serve in large shallow bowls. Combine olive oil, vinegar and lemon juice; pour over salad and toss. Place anchovies as desired on salads. You may also have decanters of olive oil and rice vinegar on the table for individuals to serve themselves in addition. Salt and ground pepper to taste. (Is this as good as it gets? I think so!).

Calories / Fat / Protein / Total Carbs-Fiber-Net Carbs / Omega 6-Omega 3 / Cholesterol

Irish chicken dinner (Serves 2 plus lunch) (378/18/41/11-6-5/4-0/120)

½ small head green cabbage (about 1 pound)	2 Tbs. olive oil
1 small onion	1 Tbs. chicken bouillon
4 carrots	Salt and pepper to taste
1 cup loosely packed spinach leaves	3 whole cloves
3 chicken breasts, skinless and boneless (6 oz each)	1 large bay leaf

Cut cabbage and onion each into 5 wedges. Cut carrots into 2 1/2-inch pieces. Heat olive oil in large pot over medium-high heat. Cook cabbage and onion wedges until lightly browned.

Add chicken pieces, carrots, beef bouillon, peppercorns, cloves, bay leaf, and 2 cups water; over high heat, heat to boiling. Reduce heat to low; cover and simmer 40 minutes, gently stirring occasionally until chicken and vegetables are tender. Add spinach before removing from heat. Stir. Serve in bowls. Save ½ servings for lunches.

Irish lamb soup Serves 2 (470/26/44/9-5-4/2-0/135)

2 Tbs. olive oil	1 medium onion, chopped
1 pound boneless lean lamb leg cut into 1-inch cubes	1 Tsp. dried thyme
3 cups water	1/4 Tsp. garlic powder
1 beef bouillon cube	1/4 Tsp. ground allspice
½ head cabbage, coarsely chopped	1/4 Tsp. pepper
3 carrots, chopped	1 bay leaf

Heat large pot with olive oil over medium-high until hot. Add lamb; cook 5 minutes or until browned. Add water and remaining ingredients; bring to a boil. Cover, reduce heat, and simmer 20 minutes or until the lamb is tender, stirring occasionally. Discard bay leaf.

Dessert

Frozen blueberries with heavy cream Serves 2 (116/5/2/15-6-9/0/15)

1 cup frozen blueberries	2 Tbs. organic heavy cream

Pour frozen blueberries into two bowls. Add 1 Tbs. of heavy cream to each bowl and stir until the berries are coated with frozen cream. This is the best iced cream you will ever have.

Breakfast

The Japanese breakfast (serves 1) (400/18/21/5-7/8-2-6/243)
Smoked fish of choice 2 oz.
Soft-boiled egg in broth of soy sauce or Miso
Small green salad with sesame oil (1 Tbs.) and rice vinegar (1 Tsp.)

Place egg in pot and cover with cold water. Turn heat on high and cook for 5 minutes. Remove egg and place in cool water. Carefully shell egg and place in small bowl with Miso soup (see recipe in soup section). May add a dash of Soy sauce if desired.

Goat cheese omelet (serves 1) (336/28/23/0/3-0/469)

2 eggs	1 Tsp. butter
1 Tbs. heavy cream	Salt and pepper to taste
1 oz. goat cheese, crumbled	

Beat eggs and cream until mixed. Melt butter in shallow pan over medium heat. Pour egg mixture into pan and swish pan to spread the egg mixture over the pan. Reduce heat to low and cook until egg is no longer runny. Spread the cheese over half of the egg mixture and flip the other half over the cheese. Cook 2-3 more minutes, flipping omelet once.

Oat bran waffles (4 servings of 2 waffles each) (339/23/10/22-2-20/160

10 almonds, unroasted	1 cup Oat-bran flour
1/3 cup Light olive oil	1 Tsp. Baking powder
1 cup spring or filtered water	3 eggs (Omega-3 enriched if available)

Put almonds in blender and blend until nuts are in powder. Now add water and blend to create almond milk. Add olive oil and eggs and blend to a smooth liquid. Pour into bowl and add remaining dry ingredients and mix well. Let sit for 5 minutes. Bake in greased waffle iron for 3 minutes per waffle. Serve with strawberries (and whipped cream?).

Topping for waffles Serves 1 (78/6/1/11-4-7/0-0/21)
4 strawberries, fresh or frozen, sliced
1 Tbs. heavy cream, plain or whipped

Calories / Fat / Protein / Total Carbs-Fiber-Net Carbs / Omega 6-Omega 3 / Cholesterol

Lunch

The Japanese lunch (130/11/9/1-5/0-0-0/30)
Sashimi tray from grocery store (buy the day before and keep in refrigerator until eaten).

Eat fish with ginger and wasabi (peel fish off and leave the rice in the tray).

Dinner

The Japanese dinner (430/29/30/6-12/8-2-6/60)
Sashimi Platter   Green salad with dressing
Miso soup

Go to your local Japanese restaurant and order their sashimi platter with Miso soup. It may also come with a spring roll (which is decadent but eat it anyway, with lots of wasabi and soy sauce).

Baked chicken breast with fresh basil Serves 4 (319/14/44/8-2-6/5-0/226)
4 boneless skinless chicken breasts (24 oz)   2 Tbs. olive oil
¼ chopped fresh basil   ½ cup oat bran
2 eggs, beaten   Salt and pepper

Pour oil into bowl and coat chicken with olive oil. Arrange in single layer in baking dish. Combine egg into olive oil; add basil and oat bran; mix well and spread over chicken.

Cover baking dish with foil and place in 375-degree oven for 30 minutes or until chicken is no longer pink inside.

Mexican chicken salad Serves 2 (296/17/25/13-5-8/1-0/80)

1 white daikon thinly sliced	2 Tbs. lime or lemon juice
8 oz. diced cooked chicken breast	1 Tsp. salt
1 medium cucumber sliced thinly and halved into crescents	½ medium head romaine lettuce, torn in 2-inch pieces
½ medium red onion thinly sliced, in crescents	¼ Tsp. chili powder
2 Tbs. olive oil	2 Tbs. coarsely chopped cilantro

Place cut up daikon in a large glass bowl. Add the chicken, cucumber and onion. In a small bowl, whisk together the oil, lime juices, and salt. Mix until blended. Pour the dressing over the chicken salad and toss to blend.

Arrange lettuce on two large salad plates. Heap half of the chicken salad on each plate. Sprinkle with the chili powder and the cilantro. Serve immediately.

Cucumber salad

2 cups cucumbers, cut in half lengthwise, seeded and chopped	2 Tsp. Fresh ginger, peeled and minced
1/2 cup carrots, grated or finely diced	1 clove garlic, finely chopped
1/4 cup scallions or red onion, finely chopped	1/2 cup water
	1/4 cup white vinegar

Combine all vegetables with ginger, garlic and crushed peppercorns in a medium or large bowl. Add vinegar and mix thoroughly. Cover and refrigerate at least 30 minutes before serving. Best if prepared a day ahead.

Black-eyed peas with garlic and kale Serves 2 (226/14/12/22-9-13/2-0/0)

1 bunch of kale washed and drained	Pinch of dried red pepper
2 Tbs. olive oil	1 cup canned or cooked black-eyed peas
1 clove garlic, pressed	1 Tbs. Cider vinegar, or to taste

Pull the kale leaves from the stems (discard stems) and chop the leaves into one inch pieces. Place about one inch of water in a large pot and heat to boiling. Add the kale, cover and cook until tender, stirring occasionally, 5 to 10 minutes. Drain. In a large non-stick skillet, combine the oil and garlic. Cook the garlic over low heat, stirring, until it begins to sizzle, about two minutes. Add the peas and red pepper and cook until blended, stirring, about three minutes. Add the kale and stir to blend over low heat. Add the cider vinegar just before serving. Serve hot or at room temperature.

Recipes for Sunday

Breakfast

Low carb waffles with blueberries Serves 6 (258/11/22/5-1/6-3-2/104)

2/3 cups almonds and walnuts with a few	1 Tsp. baking powder
Brazil nuts	1/3 cup light olive oil
1 cup filtered water	1 cup blueberries, fresh or frozen
3 organic eggs	(Whipped organic cream)
1/3 cup whey protein powder	

Put the mixed nuts and water in the blender and blend until mixture turns into nut-milk (about 3 minutes). Add eggs and olive oil and blend one minute. Pour mixture into bowl and add whey protein powder and baking powder and mix well. Put 1/3 cup of mixture in heated, greased waffle iron and cook for 3 minutes. Remove and eat immediately with blueberries (and whipped cream?). You may freeze them to eat for a quick breakfast during the week.

Western omelet Serves 2 (262/21/14/4-1-3/2-1/556)

4 eggs (organic)	¼ Tsp. dried basil
1 Tbs. fresh chives (1 Tsp. dried)	4 large mushrooms, sliced
1 Tbs. chopped green pepper	2 Tbs. Salsa
1 Tbs. chopped onion	1 Tbs. butter or olive oil

Sauté the vegetables in the butter or olive oil. Break eggs into bowl and beat until blended. Pour the vegetables onto a plate. Then add the egg mixture to the pan coating the bottom of the pan. Cover pan and cook for 1-2 min on medium heat. Add vegetable mixture and fold omelet in half. Cover pan, turn off heat and let coast turning once more. Serve hot.

Lunch

Salmon cakes Serves 1 (260/22/18/3-2-1/6-5/50)

1 7-ounce can of Salmon (3 oz dry weight)	1 Tsp. dried parsley (or 1 Tbs. fresh)
½ stalk celery, chopped	1 Tbs. Grapeseed or canola oil mayonnaise
1 Tbs. minced onion	1 Tsp. olive oil
1 clove garlic, pressed	Salt and pepper to taste

Mix all ingredients except the olive oil in a bowl and mix well. Press mixture into 2 patties. Heat olive oil (or butter) in pan and sauté cakes until they develop a crust. Then flip with a spatula. Eat warm or cold.

Crab cakes Serves 2 (190/11/9/3-2-1/0-2/50)

2 2-oz cans of crabmeat

1 egg white (discard yolk)

1 stalk celery, chopped finely

1 Tbs. minced fresh parsley

1 Tbs. Grapeseed or canola oil mayonnaise

Salt and pepper to taste

1 Tbs. olive oil

Mix all ingredients except the olive oil in a bowl and mix well. Press mixture into 2 patties. Heat olive oil (or butter) in pan and sauté cakes until they develop a crust. Then flip with a spatula. Eat warm or cold.

Shrimp salad Serves 2 (220/11/24/4-2-2/5-1/173)

2 cups cooked shrimp (8 oz)

2 Tbs. Grapeseed or canola oil mayonnaise

2 Tsp. capers

1 stalk celery, chopped

1 Tbs. Lemon juice

Freshly ground black pepper

Cut the shrimp into bite-size pieces. Place in a bowl. Add mayonnaise, capers and celery. Sprinkle lemon juice and pepper to taste over the salad. Stir to coat shrimp and blend ingredients. Serve on lettuce leaves.

Dinner

Curried chicken salad with grapes and celery Serves 4 (287/14/25/14-2-12/4-1/85)

1 lb. boiled chicken breast

4 Tbs. grape seed or canola oil mayonnaise

1-2 Tsp. curry powder (to taste)

1 Tsp. lemon juice

2 celery stalks- finely chopped

2 cups of red or green seedless grapes

Salt and pepper to taste

Mix all ingredients together. Serve with mixed green salad.

Herbed lamb chops with asparagus Serves 2 (506/30/46/13-5-8/0-0/155)

2 lamb chops ½ inches thick (6 oz. each)	1 large onion, sliced
1 Tsp. chopped fresh basil	2 cloves garlic, peeled but left whole
1 Tsp. crushed rosemary	(optional)
1 Tsp. thyme	1/3 cup dry white wine
2 Tbs. olive oil or butter	14 spears of asparagus

Heat 1Tbs. oil or butter in large skillet and sauté the onions and garlic. Discard the garlic but reserve the onion on a plate. Add remaining oil or butter and brown the lamb chops over high heat for 2 minutes on each side. Remove lamb chops to a plate. Add the spices, asparagus and wine to the skillet and heat for 3-4 minutes, scrapping up the remnants of lamb from the bottom of the pan. Return the lamb chops and onions to the pan and coat with the juices.

Beef and mushroom stew Serves 4 (293/17/18/10-2-7/0-0/125)

1 ½ pounds lean boneless organic steak	1 Tsp. chopped fresh basil
2 Tbs. olive oil	1 beef-flavored bouillon
1 large onion, sliced	½ Tsp. cracked pepper
1 clove garlic, minced	8 oz sliced fresh mushrooms
¾ cups water	¼ pound snow pea pods, trimmed and
1 Tbs. chopped fresh oregano	cut into 1-inch pieces
1 Tsp. chopped fresh parsley	

Trim fat from boneless steak, and cut steak into 1-inch pieces. Add olive oil to pot; place over medium-high heat until hot. Add steak pieces; sauté until browned on all sides, stirring frequently. Add onion and garlic; sauté until onion is tender. Stir in water, oregano, parsley, and basil. Add bouillon and pepper, stirring well. Bring to a boil; cover, reduce heat, and simmer 30-60 minutes. Add mushrooms; cover and cook 10 minutes. Add snow peas; cover and cook an additional 5 minutes or until crisp- tender.

To serve, ladle beef stew into individual serving bowls. Yield: 6 cups.

Shop the Periphery of the Grocery Store

If a Food will not Rot or Sprout
Don't eat it, but
Throw it out!

THE MEDITERRANEAN HUNTER-GATHERER

COOKBOOK

More Recipes to Get You Started

Most of the recipes from elsewhere in the book are also included in this section to save time when we are in a hurry

You are what you eat...

So watch what you eat !!!!!!!

THE MEDITERRANEAN HUNTER-GATHERER COOKBOOK

Breakfasts, Lunches and Snacks (Please see Nutrition for Women in chapter 7)

Dinner Entrees

Fish   142

Shrimp, Crab and Scallop Stew
Shrimp with Pesto
Crustless Crab and Broccoli Quiche
Crab Cakes
Salmon Cakes
Baked Haddock
Flounder Creole
Sautéed Flounder
Flounder Fillets with Shrimp
Indian Grilled Shrimp
Salmon Fillets with Lemon and Garlic
Salmon Fillets with Mustard and Mayo Glaze

Poultry   147

Irish Chicken Dinner
Baked Chicken with Fresh Basil
Curried Turkey
Chicken with Cinnamon-Raisin Sauce
Habañero Chicken
Chicken Stew
Chicken Stir-Fry

Beef and Lamb   150

Filet Mignon (or other lean steak) with sautéed onions
Broiled Lamb Kebobs
Beef and Mushroom Stew
Italian Pot Roast
Calabrian Beef Stew

Vegetables

Asparagus with Lemon
Sautéed Sweet Peppers, Leeks and Rosemary
Greens with Garlic and olive oil or other fat
California style broccoli with mayonnaise (canola or grape seed oil)
Zucchini and Onion Sautéed
Cauliflower with Ginger
Sprout and Snow Pea Stir-Fry
Roasted Vegetables
Brussel Sprouts
Spinach
Collard Greens
Broccoli
Mixed Winter Vegetables
Cauliflower
Black-Eyed Peas with Garlic and Kale
Okra with Stewed Tomatoes
Turkey and Avocado Lettuce Wrap

Soups

Miso Soup
Hearty Salmon Chowder
Cabbage Soup
Irish Lamb Soup

Salads

Green Leafy/Vegetarian

Renaissance Greek Salad
Curried Salad
Spinach and Red Cabbage Salad
Black Bean Salad
Piquant Vegetable Salad
Cucumber Salad
Spinach Salad
St. Patrick's Shamrock Salad

Beef Burritos and Salad

Chinese Chicken with Broccoli and Peanuts

Meat/Fish/Poultry Salads

Tuna Salad

Chicken Salad

Shrimp, crab and scallop stew (Serves 2 plus two 1/3 cup lunch servings) (407/17/48/13-3-10/2-3/285)

2 Tbs. olive oil

½ Cup chopped onion

1 clove garlic, minced

7 oz can of whole tomatoes, undrained and chopped

¼ Cup chopped fresh oregano

2 Tbs. chopped fresh parsley

1 Tsp. low-sodium Worcestershire sauce

1/8 Tsp. red pepper

½ pound bay scallops (fresh or frozen)

½ pound medium-size shrimp, peeled and de-veined (fresh or frozen)

2 oz. can of white crab meat

Add the olive oil to the pot; place over medium-high heat until hot. Add chopped onion, sweet red pepper, add minced garlic; sauté until vegetables are tender. Add tomato, stirring well to combine. Add oregano and next 3 ingredients; stir well. Bring vegetable mixture to a boil over medium heat; cover, reduce heat, and simmer 20 minutes. Add scallops and shrimp to vegetable mixture; bring to a boil. Reduce heat, and simmer 7 to 8 minutes or until scallops and shrimp are done.

Shrimp with pesto Serves 2 (568/35/42/3-2-1/5-2/260)

12 oz fresh or frozen shrimp

1 cup fresh basil

1 large garlic clove, pressed

¼ cup olive oil

1 Tbs. grated Parmesan cheese

Add basil, garlic and olive oil to blender and blend on medium-high until basil is completely chopped and mixed with olive oil. Add Parmesan cheese and blend until mix. Let set while cooking shrimp.

Boil water in medium pot, add shrimp and cook for 3-4 minutes for fresh shrimp or 4-6 minutes for frozen shrimp. Drain shrimp and place in bowl. Pour pesto sauce over the shrimp, stir and serve immediately or may keep in refrigerator to serve later.

Crustless crab and broccoli quiche Serves 6 (136/8/12/4-2-2/1-1/245)

1 Tbs. olive oil

1 cup chopped fresh broccoli

½ cup finely chopped sweet red pepper

¼ cup finely chopped onion

¼ cup water

4 large eggs, lightly beaten

1 (6-ounce) can lump crabmeat, drained

½ cup almond milk

½ Tsp. salt

¼ Tsp. dry mustard

¼ Tsp. ground red pepper

Combine broccoli, sweet red pepper, onion, and olive oil in a medium saucepan. Cover and cook over medium heat 3 to 5 minutes or until vegetables are crisp-tender. Combine vegetable mixture, beaten eggs and next 6 ingredients in a large bowl, stirring well. Pour mixture into a 9-inch quiche dish coated with cooking spray. Bake at 350° for 35 to 40 minutes or until set. Let stand 10 minutes before slicing into 6 wedges.

Crab cakes Serves 2 (190/11/9/3-2-1/0-2/50)

2 2-oz cans of crabmeat

1 egg white (discard yolk)

1 stalk celery, chopped finely

1 Tbs. minced fresh parsley

1 Tbs. Grapeseed or canola oil mayonnaise

Salt and pepper to taste

1 Tbs. olive oil

Mix all ingredients except the olive oil in a bowl and mix well. Press mixture into 2 patties. Heat olive oil (or butter) in pan and sauté cakes until they develop a crust. Then flip with a spatula. Eat warm or cold.

Salmon cakes Serves 1 (260/22/18/3-2-1/6-5/50)

1 7-ounce can of Salmon (3 oz dry weight)

½ stalk celery, chopped

1 Tbs. minced onion

1 clove garlic, pressed

1 Tsp. dried parsley (or 1 Tbs. fresh)

1 Tbs. Grapeseed or canola oil mayonnaise

1 Tsp. olive oil

Salt and pepper to taste

Mix all ingredients except the olive oil in a bowl and mix well. Press mixture into 2 patties. Heat olive oil (or butter) in pan and sauté cakes until they develop a crust. Then flip with a spatula. Eat warm or cold.

Calories / Fat / Protein / Total Carbs-Fiber-Net Carbs / Omega 6-Omega 3 / Cholesterol

Baked haddock Serves 4
Calories 215, Fat 10, Mono 7, Poly 1/1, Sat 1, Carbohydrate 9, Sugar 4, Fiber 3, Protein 21

1 pound fresh or frozen haddock fillets,
2 Tbs. Lemon juice
1-2 cloves garlic, crushed
4 green onions with tops, chopped
1 stalk celery, chopped
2 Tbs. olive oil
1/4 cup dry white wine

2 tomatoes, peeled and chopped (11 oz can or 2 fresh)
1/8 Tsp. red and black pepper
2 parsley sprigs, chopped
5 fresh basil leaves, minced (or 1/2 Tsp. dried)
Lemon wedges

Allow haddock fillets to stand at room temperature 30-60 minutes (if frozen). Preheat oven to 425 degrees. Sauté green onions, celery and garlic in olive oil in large skillet over medium heat for 3 minutes. Add wine, chopped tomatoes, parsley, and basil. Simmer uncovered over medium heat, stirring occasionally until thickened (about 20 minutes).

Cut fish into 8 portions of equal thickness, cutting on a slant. Place into a baking pan just large enough to fit portions. Cover with mixture of lemon juice and pepper. Bake fish 15 minutes uncovered. Remove from oven and pour sauce over fish. Reduce oven to 350 degrees and bake fish 5 to 8 minutes longer, or until fish becomes opaque.

Flounder Creole Serves 2 (340/19/30/12-2-10/2-5/100)

Flounder fillets 1 lb.
2 Tbs. olive oil
½ red onion, chopped
2 cloves garlic, crushed
7 oz can of whole tomatoes, undrained and chopped

1 Tbs. Worcestershire sauce
1 Tbs. rice vinegar
3/4 Tsp. dried basil
1/4 Tsp. salt
Pinch ground red pepper

Heat oil in large skillet or wok over medium heat. Add onion and garlic and sauté until tender. Add tomato and remaining ingredients except fish. Bring to a boil. Add fillets, spooning tomato mixture over fish. Reduce heat, cover and simmer 12 minutes.

Calories / Fat / Protein / Total Carbs-Fiber-Net Carbs / Omega 6-Omega 3 / Cholesterol

Sautéed flounder Serves 2 (320/13/38/6-2-4/1-2/100)

1 lb. Flounder fillet	¼ Tsp. red pepper
1 medium onion, sliced	Salt to taste
2 Tbs. fresh parsley, chopped finely	Dash of soy sauce
1 Tbs. organic butter or olive oil	

Heat heavy skillet until hot. Add butter and onion, reduce heat and sauté until limp (1-2 minutes). Add fillet and cook the first side until fish is no longer translucent (3-4 minutes). Turn and cook second side as the first. Cover and turn off heat. Let sit for 3-5 minutes. The fish will be easy to pull apart with a fork when done.

Flounder fillet with shrimp Serves 2 (285/10/46/3-2-1/2-1/162)

2 onion slices	4 flounder fillets (4 ounces each)
1 Tsp. lemon juice	Salt and freshly ground black pepper
2 parsley sprigs	¼ pound mushrooms, sliced
1 bay leaf	1 cup water
¼ Tsp. ground thyme	1 Tbs. olive oil
12 small shrimp, shelled and deveined (4 oz)	

Preheat oven to 325° F. Sauté the mushrooms and onion slices in the olive oil. Add the lemon juice, parsley, bay leaf, thyme, and water. Bring mixture to a boil. Add the shrimp, and cook them for three to five minutes.

Place the flounder fillets in a double layer in a two-inch-deep baking dish, seasoning between the layers with salt and pepper. Pour the sauce over the fish, cover and bake for fifteen to twenty minutes or until the fish flakes easily when tested with a fork. Garnish with shrimp and place under the broiler until lightly browned and hot.

Indian grilled shrimp Serves 4 (280/10/26/6-3-3/2-1/320)

16 oz. Shrimp, peeled and deveined	1 Tsp. Ground turmeric
1 1/2 Tbs. Lemon or lime juice	1/4 Tsp. Ground cumin
2 Tbs. olive oil	1 cup wild rice
3 garlic cloves, crushed through a press	2 cups water
1 1/2-Tsp. Fresh thyme leaves (or 3/4 Tsp. Dried)	1/2 Tsp. Salt
1/4-1/2 Tsp. Crushed red pepper (or to taste)	

Toss shrimp with lime juice, garlic, thyme and red pepper. Cover and marinate at least one hour. When ready to cook, start with the rice. Place turmeric, cumin and rice in a skillet and heat over low heat, just until fragrant (about 30 seconds). Add water and salt.

Heat to boiling, then cover and cook over low heat until water is absorbed and rice is tender (about 15 minutes).

Prepare shrimp when rice is almost done; cook quickly in olive oil until lightly browned on both sides. Spoon rice onto a platter and top with shrimp.

Salmon fillets with lemon and garlic Serves 4 (337/25/18/10-1-9/6-4/168)

1 lb. Salmon fillet, cut into 4 equal pieces	I red onion, cut lengthwise into thin slices
¾ cup extra-virgin olive oil	
½ cup fresh orange juice	4 or 5 cloves garlic, pressed
Juice of 1 lemon	I (1-inch) piece ginger root, thinly sliced
4 to 5 Tbs. soy sauce	½ Tsp. chili powder

Place salmon in a shallow baking dish. For marinade, combine remaining ingredients in a medium bowl. Pour marinade over salmon. Marinate in the refrigerator 2 to 3 hours, occasionally spooning marinade over salmon.

Preheat broiler. Drain salmon, reserving marinade. Place salmon on foil in broiler pan. Broil, brushing frequently with marinade, until browned on the topside, about 3 minutes. Turn and broil until the salmon is just opaque in the center, about 3 minutes. Transfer to a serving platter and serve immediately.

Salmon fillets with mustard and mayonnaise glaze Serves 2 & 2 lunches (492/37/36/2-0-2/17-9/93)

1 lb. Salmon fillet, cut into 4 equal pieces	1 Tbs. lemon juice
4 Tbs. Grape seed oil mayonnaise	4 or 5 cloves garlic, pressed
2 Tbs. spicy mustard	

Place salmon in a shallow baking dish. Blend remaining ingredients together in a bowl and spread evenly over top of salmon fillets. Place under heated broiler for 5 minutes. Turn off oven keeping oven door closed and let "coast" for an additional 5-10 minutes or until the salmon is just opaque in the center. Transfer to a serving platter and serve immediately.

Irish chicken dinner Serves 2 plus lunch (378/18/41/11-6-5/4-0/120)

½ small head green cabbage (about 1 pound)	2 Tbs. olive oil
1 small onion	1 Tbs. chicken bouillon
4 carrots	Salt and pepper to taste
1 cup loosely packed spinach leaves	3 whole cloves
3 chicken breasts, skinless and boneless (6 oz each)	1 large bay leaf

Cut cabbage and onion each into 5 wedges. Cut carrots into 2 1/2-inch pieces. Heat olive oil in large pot over medium-high heat. Cook cabbage and onion wedges until lightly browned.

Add chicken pieces, carrots, chicken bouillon, peppercorns, cloves, bay leaf, and 2 cups water; over high heat, heat to boiling. Reduce heat to low; cover and simmer 40 minutes, gently stirring occasionally until chicken and vegetables are tender. Add spinach before removing from heat. Stir. Serve in bowls. Save ½ servings for lunches.

Baked chicken breast with fresh basil Serves 4 (319/14/44/8-2-6/5-0/226)

4 boneless skinless chicken breasts (24 oz)	2 Tbs. olive oil
¼ chopped fresh basil	½ cup oat bran
2 eggs, beaten	Salt and pepper

Pour oil into bowl and coat chicken with olive oil. Arrange in single layer in baking dish. Combine egg into olive oil; add basil and oat bran; mix well and spread over chicken.

Cover baking dish with foil and place in 375-degree oven for 30 minutes or until chicken is no longer pink inside.

Curried turkey Serves 4 (295/12/32/6-2-4/5-0/180)

1 lb. turkey breast cut into cubes	1-2 Tsp. Curry powder
1 Tbs. parsley flakes	1/4 to 1/2 Tsp. Ginger
1/8 Tsp. Pepper	1/8 Tsp. Ground cloves
2 Tbs. olive oil	1 cup chicken broth or bouillon
1/2 cup minced onion	1 Tsp. Lemon juice
1 tart apple	

Brown turkey and onion in olive oil in a skillet. Add parsley and pepper. While turkey cooks, mince apple into small pieces. Add onion, apple, curry and ginger. Cook, stirring occasionally, until onion and apple are transparent. Blend in liquid and cook, stirring, until mixture comes to a full rolling boil. Add lemon juice and stir. Serve in bowls.

Chicken with cinnamon-raisin sauce Serves 4

Calories 370, Fat 13, Poly 0/5, Sat 4, Carbohydrate 12, Sugar 9, Fiber 2, Protein 54

2 Tsp. olive oil	4 boneless chicken breast halves (6 oz each)
1/2 cup chopped onion	
3/4 Tsp. cinnamon	1 Tbs. lemon juice
1/8 Tsp. fresh ground pepper	1/4 cup raisins
3 cloves garlic, minced	

Heat olive oil briefly in large skillet; add onion, cinnamon, pepper and garlic. Cook over medium-high heat for 3-4 minutes, stirring frequently to prevent sticking. Add chicken and cook about 5 minutes on each side.

Add lemon juice and raisins, cover, and simmer over low heat about 10 minutes more. When chicken is done, serve chicken with some of the onion-raisin mixture spooned on top.

Habañero chicken Serves 4

1 cup diced onion	1 Tsp. Ground allspice
3 scallions, green and white parts, chopped	½ Tsp. Freshly ground black pepper
2 Tbs. Fresh thyme leaves, or 2 Tsp. Dried	½ Tsp. Ground cinnamon
1 Tbs. Coarsely chopped gingerroot	¼ Tsp. Freshly ground nutmeg
2 Habañero Chile peppers or ½ Tsp. Red pepper	½ Tsp. Salt
1 Tbs. olive oil	2 chicken breasts, split and skinned

Preheat the oven to 300 F. In a blender, combine the onion, scallion, thyme, ginger, chiles or red pepper, oil, allspice, pepper, cinnamon, nutmeg and salt. Process to a pulpy paste. There will be about a cup. Spread the paste liberally over the chicken breasts. Place the chicken in a baking dish, cover and bake 45 minutes or until chicken is done.

Chicken stew Serves 4

Calories 304, Fat 12, Poly 0/3, Sat 3, Carbohydrate 13, Sugar 3, Fiber 2, Protein 36

4 (4-ounce) skinned, boned organic chicken breast halves

2 Tbs. olive oil

1 cup thinly sliced green onions

½ cup sliced onion

4 cloves garlic, minced

2-14.5 oz cans diced tomatoes with Italian herbs

1 cup dry white wine

1 bay leaf

1 Tsp. dried whole thyme

½ Tsp. fennel seeds, crushed

¼ Tsp. salt

1/8 Tsp. saffron powder (optional)

Dash of ground red pepper

Freshly ground pepper (optional)

Heat olive oil in a pot over medium-high heat until hot. Add onions and garlic; sauté until onion is tender. Add chicken, diced tomatoes with Italian herbs, wine, and bay leaf to onion mixture, stirring well to combine. Add thyme, fennel seeds, salt, saffron, and red pepper and bring to boil stirring well.

Reduce heat, cover, and simmer 20-25 minutes or until done. Remove and discard bay leaf. Ladle stew into individual bowls, and garnish with freshly ground pepper, if desired.

Chicken stir-fry Serves 2 (360/13/54/6-2-4/5-0/120)

12 oz Chicken breast cut into 1/2-inch-wide strips

1 Tbs. olive oil

1 medium onion, sliced

1 clove garlic, minced

1 Tsp. curry powder

½ Tsp. salt

½ Tsp. dried thyme

1/8 Tsp. ground red pepper

2 Tbs. chopped fresh parsley

Add olive oil and chicken to skillet. Stir-fry over medium-high heat for 3 minutes or until lightly browned. Add onion and garlic; stir-fry 3 minutes or until tender. Add curry powder and next 4 ingredients; stir well. Reduce heat. Simmer for 10-15 minutes or until tender. Spoon into bowls and sprinkle with parsley.

BEEF AND LAMB

Filet mignon (or other lean steak) with sautéed onions Serves1 plus 1 breakfast
(338/27/48/6-2-4/3-0/130)

8 oz filet mignon	1 Tbs. Organic butter
1 medium onion, sliced	Salt and pepper to taste
½ pound mushrooms, sliced	

Heat heavy skillet until hot. Add butter, mushrooms and onion and sauté until limp (1-2 minutes). Add filet and sear the first side until brown (1-2 minutes). Turn and sear second side as the first. Cover and turn off heat. Let sit for 3-5 minutes. The steak will be rare or medium rare, depending on the thickness. You may cook longer if you desire.

Broiled lamb kebobs Serves 4
Calories 350, Fat 19, Mono 8, Poly 0/3, Sat 8, Carbohydrate 8, Sugar 2, Fiber 3, Protein 36

1 lb. Boneless lamb loin	Salt and freshly ground pepper to taste
2 Tbs. olive oil	8 small onions, peeled
2 Tbs. Lemon juice	1 small red pepper
1 Tsp. Oregano	1 small yellow or green pepper

Cut the lamb into 1-inch cubes. Place the cubes in a glass dish and sprinkle with lemon juice, oregano, and salt and pepper to taste. Peel the onions and sauté the whole onions in olive oil 10 to 15 minutes or until almost tender. Seed the peppers and cut them into 1 1/2-inch pieces.

Thread the lamb alternating with vegetables onto flat-bladed metal skewers or wooden skewers that have been soaked in water.

Preheat the broiler. Place the skewers on a broiling pan and cook about 5 inches from the heat, turning every 3 to 4 minutes, for 12 minutes or until meat is brown outside but still pink inside.

Calories / Fat / Protein / Total Carbs-Fiber-Net Carbs / Omega 6-Omega 3 / Cholesterol

Beef and mushroom stew Serves 4 (293/17/18/10-2-7/0-0/125)

1 ½ pounds lean boneless organic steak	1 Tsp. chopped fresh basil
2 Tbs. olive oil	1 beef-flavored bouillon
1 large onion, sliced	½ Tsp. cracked pepper
1 clove garlic, minced	8 oz sliced fresh mushrooms
¾ cups water	¼ pound snow pea pods, trimmed and
1 Tbs. chopped fresh oregano	cut into 1-inch pieces
1 Tsp. chopped fresh parsley	

Trim fat from boneless steak, and cut steak into 1-inch pieces. Add olive oil to pot; place over medium-high heat until hot. Add steak pieces; sauté until browned on all sides, stirring frequently. Add onion and garlic; sauté until onion is tender. Stir in water, oregano, parsley, and basil. Add bouillon and pepper, stirring well. Bring to a boil; cover, reduce heat, and simmer 30-60 minutes. Add mushrooms; cover and cook 10 minutes. Add snow peas; cover and cook an additional 5 minutes or until crisp- tender.

To serve, ladle beef stew into individual serving bowls.

Italian pot roast Serves 2 plus 2 lunches (600/46/60/12-5-7/0-0/180)

1 lb. organic beef roast cut into 2-inch cubes	½ Tsp. thyme
¼ lb. Hot organic Italian sausage	½ Tsp. oregano
1 medium onion, chopped	1 Tsp. basil
3 garlic cloves, pressed	½ Tsp. cayenne pepper
2 carrots cut into 1 inch pieces	1/8-Tsp. fennel seeds
4 celery stalks, cut into 1 inch pieces	2 Tbs. olive oil
1 red pepper, chopped	1 Tbs. organic butter
12 mushrooms, sliced	2 Tbs. organic heavy cream
2 Tbs. fresh chopped parsley	1 cup water

Heat olive oil and butter in large pot. Sauté beef and sausage for 5 minutes or until browned. Add onion and garlic and sauté for additional 5 minutes. Add remaining ingredients, bring to boil, cover and reduce heat and simmer for 1-1/2 to 2 hours or until beef is tender. Serve in bowls.

Calabrian beef stew Serves 4

Calories 253, Fat 17, Mono 5, Poly 1/5, Sat 6, Carbohydrate 7, Sugar 3, Fiber 2, Protein 18

1 ½ pounds lean boneless organic round steak (1/2-inch thick)

2 Tbs. olive oil

1 large onion, sliced

1 clove garlic, minced

¾ cups water

½ cup balsamic vinegar

1 Tbs. chopped fresh oregano

1 Tsp. chopped fresh parsley

1 Tsp. chopped fresh basil

2 Tsp. beef-flavored bouillon granules

½ Tsp. cracked pepper

2 medium-size sweet red peppers cut into 1-inch pieces

2 medium-size sweet yellow peppers, cut into 1-inch pieces

1 cup sliced fresh mushrooms

¼ pound snow pea pods, trimmed and cut into 1-inch pieces

Trim fat from boneless round steak, and cut steak into 1-inch pieces. Add olive oil to pot; place over medium-high heat until hot. Add steak pieces; sauté until browned on all sides, stirring frequently. Add onion and garlic; sauté until onion is tender. Stir in water, vinegar, oregano, parsley, and basil. Add bouillon granules and pepper, stirring well. Bring to a boil; cover, reduce heat, and simmer 1 hour. Add pepper pieces and mushrooms; cover and cook 10 minutes. Add snow peas; cover and cook an additional 5 minutes or until crisp- tender.

To serve, ladle beef stew into individual serving bowls.

Asparagus with lemon Serves 2 (60/0/6/12-4-8/0)

14 spears of asparagus

1 Tsp. butter

1 Tbs. water

1 Tbs. lemon juice

Place all ingredients in skillet and heat to steaming. Cover and simmer on low for 4-6 minutes. Remove from heat and serve immediately on a warm plate.

Sautéed sweet peppers, leeks and rosemary Serves 2

4 small leeks

1 small green zucchini (summer squash)

2 sweet peppers (red, yellow)

1 sprig fresh rosemary or 1 Tsp. dried

2 Tbs. olive oil

Salt and pepper

Trim all but 1-inch of green from leeks; wash under cold water. In saucepan of boiling water, cook leeks for 5 minutes or until tender and then drain.

Cut zucchini into 1/2-inch thick diagonal slices. Clean peppers and cut into strips. Remove leaves from rosemary. Sauté peppers, zucchini, leeks and rosemary in olive oil over medium heat stirring occasionally, for 5 to 10 minutes or until tender. Season with salt and pepper to taste. Arrange on warm serving platter.

Greens with garlic and olive oil or other fat Serves 2

2 Tbs. extra-virgin olive oil

1 small leek, white part only, sliced

3 scallions, chopped, green and white parts

2 large cloves garlic, crushed in press

3 cups chopped kale from garden

3 cups chopped broccoli rape or 10-oz package frozen, defrosted

2 cups collards cut in 1/2-inch ribbons or 10-oz package frozen, defrosted

3 cups fresh spinach or 10-oz. Package frozen, defrosted

½ cup water

Freshly ground pepper to taste

Heat the oil in a large skillet over medium-high heat. Add the leek, scallions and garlic. Sauté until the leeks are limp, about 4 minutes. Add the kale, broccoli rape, and collards, stirring until they are wilted. Mix in the spinach. Add the water and simmer until the greens are tender, about 5-10 minutes, stirring occasionally, season to taste with salt and pepper. Remove from heat and add olive oil and stir to mix. Serve immediately.

California style broccoli with grape seed oil mayonnaise Serves 2
(175/11/9/12-6-6/3-0/0)
1 lb. broccoli (12 spears)
2 Tbs. grape seed oil mayonnaise

Steam broccoli for 3-5 minutes. Serve immediately with topping of mayonnaise.

Zucchini and onion sautéed Serves 2

4 small zucchini, sliced 1/4 inch thick
1 medium onion, sliced into 1/4 inch wedges
3 Tbs. olive oil

1 clove garlic, crushed in a press
1/4 Tsp. red and black pepper

Add olive oil to skillet; cook the zucchini and onion over medium heat. Add the remaining ingredients and cook on low heat for 3 minutes or until the zucchini has reached a desired tenderness.

Cauliflower with ginger Serves 2

1 small head cauliflower, chopped into 1 to 1 1/2-inch florets (about 4 cups)
1/4 cup hot water
2 Tbs. light olive oil
1/2 Tsp. cumin

1 Tbs. fresh gingerroot, minced
1/2 Tsp. turmeric
2 Tsp. lemon juice
1 Tbs. fresh coriander leaves, chopped

Heat a large skillet over medium-high heat about 30 seconds; add oil and heat another 30 seconds. Add cumin, ginger and turmeric and stir to mix, then immediately add cauliflower and stir again to distribute spices. Add water, reduce heat, cover and cook until the cauliflower is crisp-tender (about 10 minutes). Stir gently once part way through cooking. When cauliflower is almost ready, remove cover, increase heat to medium and gently stir-fry to evaporate any moisture and lightly brown cauliflower. Add lemon juice and chopped coriander, toss lightly and serve immediately.

Sprout and snow pea stir-fry Serves 2

4 cups snow peas (8 oz)

1 Tsp. Toasted Sesame oil

2 Tsp. minced garlic

2 Tbs. minced gingerroot

2 cups bean sprouts (4-oz/125 g)

3 Tbs. water (optional)

2 Tsp. soy sauce

Remove stem end and string from snow peas. In large nonstick skillet or wok, heat oil over high heat. Add garlic, gingerroot and snow peas; stir-fry for 1 minute. Add bean sprouts; stir-fry for 1 minute or until vegetables are tender-crisp. Stir in soy sauce.

Roasted vegetables Serves 2

3 Tbs. Balsamic or red wine vinegar

2 Tbs. olive oil

1/4-cup fresh basil, chopped or 1 Tbs. dried

1 small eggplant, sliced into thin rounds

1 zucchini, thinly sliced

1 yellow summer squash, thinly sliced

1 red bell pepper, seeded and sliced thinly

1 small red onion, sliced and separated

Preheat oven to 450 degrees. Blend vinegar, oil and basil. Add vegetables, tossing to coat. Place vegetables in roasting pan and cook, stirring occasionally, until tender and lightly browned – about 30 minutes. Cool vegetables.

Brussel sprouts, steamed with olive oil, red and black pepper (garlic optional) Serves 2

Calories 200, Fat 14, Poly 0/2, Sat 2, Carbohydrate 10, Sugar 5, Fiber 5, Protein 6

12 oz frozen or fresh Brussel sprouts

2 Tbs. olive oil

Red and black pepper to taste

1 clove garlic, pressed (optional)

Bring ¼ cup water to boil in a medium saucepan. Add the Brussel sprouts (and garlic if desired) and steam at medium heat for 3-5 minutes or until warm (if using fresh, steam for 12-15 minutes or until cooked). Remove from heat and add remaining ingredients stirring well. Serve immediately.

Spinach, steamed with olive oil, red and black pepper, and soy sauce (garlic optional)
Serves 2
Calories 170, Fat 14, Mono 10, Poly 0/2, Sat 2, Carbohydrate 4, Sugar 1, Fiber 3, Protein 4

12 oz of frozen or fresh spinach	1 Tbs. soy sauce
2 Tbs. olive oil	1 clove garlic, pressed (optional)
Red and black pepper to taste	

Bring ¼ cup water to boil in a medium saucepan. Add the spinach (and garlic if desired) and steam at medium heat for 3-5 minutes or until warm (if using fresh, steam for 8-10 minutes or until limp). Remove from heat and add remaining ingredients stirring well. Serve immediately.

Collard Greens, steamed with olive oil, red and black pepper, and soy sauce (garlic optional) Serves 2
Calories 170, Fat 14, Mono 10, Poly 0/2, Sat 2, Carbohydrate 4, Sugar 1, Fiber 3, Protein 4

12 oz of frozen or fresh collard greens	1Tbs. soy sauce
2 Tbs. olive oil	1 clove garlic, pressed (optional)
Red and black pepper to taste	

Bring ¼ cup water to boil in a medium saucepan. Add the greens (and garlic if desired) and steam at medium heat for 3-5 minutes or until warm (if using fresh, steam for 8-10 minutes or until limp). Remove from heat and add remaining ingredients stirring well. Serve immediately.

Broccoli, steamed with olive oil, red and black pepper, and soy sauce (garlic optional)
Serves 2
Calories 180, Fat 14, Mono 10, Poly 0/2, Sat 2, Carbohydrate 8, Sugar 2, Fiber 4, Protein 6

12 oz of frozen or fresh broccoli	1Tbs. soy sauce
2 Tbs. olive oil	1 clove garlic, pressed (optional)
Red and black pepper to taste	

Bring ¼ cup water to boil in a medium saucepan. Add the broccoli (and garlic if desired) and steam at medium heat for 3-5 minutes or until warm (if using fresh, steam for 8-10 minutes). Remove from heat and add remaining ingredients stirring well. Serve immediately.

Mixed Winter Vegetables, steamed with olive oil, red and black pepper, and soy sauce (garlic optional) Serves 2

Calories 180, Fat 14, Poly 0/2, Sat 2, Carbohydrate 10, Sugar 4, Fiber 4, Protein 4

12 oz of frozen or fresh mixed winter vegetables (broccoli, cauliflower, carrots)	Red and black pepper to taste
	1 Tbs. soy sauce
2 Tbs. olive oil	1 clove garlic, pressed (optional)

Bring ¼ cup water to boil in a medium saucepan. Add the vegetables (and garlic if desired) and steam at medium heat for 3-5 minutes or until warm (if using fresh, steam for 8-10 minutes). Remove from heat and add remaining ingredients stirring well. Serve immediately.

Cauliflower, steamed with olive oil, garlic, red and black pepper, and soy sauce Serves 2

Calories 180, Fat 14, Poly 0/2, Sat 2, Carbohydrate 10, Sugar 2, Fiber 4, Protein 6

12 oz of frozen or fresh cauliflower	1Tbs. soy sauce
2 Tbs. olive oil	1 clove garlic, pressed (optional)
Red and black pepper to taste	

Bring ¼ cup water to boil in a medium saucepan. Add the cauliflower (and garlic if desired) and steam at medium heat for 3-5 minutes or until warm (if using fresh, steam for 8-10 minutes). Remove from heat and add remaining ingredients stirring well. Serve immediately.

Black-eyed peas with garlic and kale Serves 2

Calories 290, Fat 14, Poly 0/2, Sat 2, Carbohydrate 22, Sugar 4, Fiber 9, Protein 12

12 oz kale (4 cups), washed and drained	Pinch of dried red pepper
2 Tbs. olive oil	1 cup canned or cooked black-eyed peas
1 clove garlic, pressed	1 Tbs. cider vinegar, or to taste

Pull the kale leaves from the stems (discard stems) and chop the leaves into one inch pieces. Place about one inch of water in a large pot and heat to boiling. Add the kale, cover and cook until tender, stirring occasionally, 5 to 10 minutes. Drain. Reserve the water for soup, if desired. In a large non-stick skillet, combine the oil and garlic. Cook the garlic over low heat, stirring, until it begins to sizzle, about two minutes. Add the peas and red pepper and cook until blended, stirring, about three minutes. Add the kale and stir to blend over low heat. Add the cider vinegar just before serving. Serve hot or at room temperature.

Okra with stewed tomatoes Serves 2

2 Tbs. olive oil

1/2 cup coarsely chopped onion

1 cup (about 1/4 pound) fresh (or frozen) okra cut in 3/4-inch pieces

8 oz. can stewed tomatoes

Freshly ground pepper to taste

In a deep saucepan, heat the oil over medium high heat. Sauté the onion until it softens, about 4 minutes. Add the okra and sauté 3 to 4 minutes, until it turns bright green. Add the tomatoes, bring to a boil, reduce the heat, and simmer until the okra is crisp-tender, about 5 minutes. Season to taste with pepper. Serve immediately.

Turkey and avocado lettuce wrap Serves 1

1 large leaf Romaine lettuce

2 oz. thinly sliced turkey breast

2 Tbs. chunky salsa, well drained

1 Tsp. minced cilantro

2 1/2-inch wedges avocado

Lay the Romaine lettuce leaf on a cutting board. Cover half with sliced turkey. Spread the salsa over the turkey. Sprinkle with cilantro. Place the avocado wedges across the turkey. Fold the lettuce up over the avocado. Eat carefully over plate.

SOUPS

Miso soup Serves 2

3 cups spring or filtered water

3/4 to 1 ½ Tsp. brown rice Miso

3 (1 inch) pieces wakame or other seaweed cut up

Green onions, thinly sliced

Several pieces each of a few vegetables such as:-onion slices-daikon matchsticks-carrot rounds-finely shredded

Chinese cabbage or head cabbage-diced winter squash

Add all ingredients except Miso to water and heat to boiling. Reduce heat and simmer 3-5 minutes. Remove from heat and allow cooling for 1-2 minutes, then add Miso and serve.

Hearty salmon chowder Serves 2

1 can (7 1/2 oz.) salmon
1 Tbs. olive oil
1/2 cup each chopped onion and celery
1/4 chopped sweet green pepper
1 clove garlic, minced
1 cup diced carrots

1 cup each chicken stock and water
1/2 Tsp. each coarse pepper and dill seed
2 cup diced zucchini
Pepper
1/2 cup chopped fresh parsley (optional)

Drain and flake salmon, reserving liquid. In large nonstick saucepan, heat olive oil over medium heat; cook onion, celery, green pepper and garlic, stirring often, for 5 minutes or until vegetables are tender.

Add carrots, chicken stock, water, pepper and dill seed; bring to boil. Reduce heat, cover and simmer for 20 minutes or until vegetables are tender. Add zucchini; simmer, covered, for 5 minutes.

Add salmon, reserving liquid, and pepper to taste. Cook over low heat just until heated through. Just before serving, add parsley.

Cabbage soup Serves 4

1 Tbs. canola oil
2 medium onions, chopped
1 medium carrot, grated
1 medium leek, white part only, chopped
1/3 small head cabbage, quartered and sliced crosswise into 1/2-inch strips, about 6 cups
4 cups vegetable stock or canned broth

1/2 cup oatmeal, steel-cut or old-fashioned
1 Tsp. dried thyme
1/2 Tsp. sugar
1 bay leaf
1/2 Tsp. salt
Freshly ground pepper

Heat the oil in a large Dutch oven or saucepan over medium-high heat. Add the onion, carrot and leek and stir to coat with the oil. Cover the pot tightly, reduce the heat to medium, and cook the vegetables for 10 minutes. Mix in the cabbage, cover the pot, and cook for another 10 minutes, until the cabbage is wilted.

Stir in the tomatoes, stock, oatmeal, thyme, sugar, bay leaf and salt. Season the soup to taste with pepper and simmer, uncovered, until the oatmeal is cooked and the cabbage is tender. This should take about 30 minutes if using steel-cut oats, and 20 minutes if using rolled oats. Serve, or cool and refrigerate overnight. When reheating, to regain a soup-like consistency, you may want to add some vegetable broth.

Irish lamb soup Serves 2 (470/26/44/9-5-4/2-0/135)

2 Tbs. olive oil

1 pound boneless lean lamb leg cut into 1-inch cubes

3 cups water

1 beef bouillon cube

½ head cabbage, coarsely chopped

3 carrots, chopped

1 medium onion, chopped

1 Tsp. dried thyme

1/4 Tsp. garlic powder

1/4 Tsp. ground allspice

1/4 Tsp. pepper

1 bay leaf

Heat olive oil in large pot over medium-high until hot. Add lamb; cook 5 minutes or until browned. Add water and remaining ingredients; bring to a boil. Cover, reduce heat, and simmer 20 minutes or until the lamb is tender, stirring occasionally. Discard bay leaf.

SALADS   Green Leafy/Vegetarian

Renaissance Greek salad Serves 2 (600/50/18/20-6-14/2-0/44)

4 cups (6 oz) mixed greens or lettuce

12 mushrooms, quartered

1 large tomato, chopped

1 green pepper, chopped

¼ Bermuda onion, thinly sliced

10 black olives (pitted or non-pitted)

½ cucumber, sliced thinly

4 oz. Feta (goat) cheese, crumbled

¼ cup olive oil

1 Tbs. lemon juice

1 Tbs. rice vinegar

½ Tsp. oregano leaves

Salt and pepper to taste

Optional: 1 small can of anchovies

Mix salad ingredients and serve in large shallow bowls. Combine olive oil, vinegar and lemon juice; pour over salad and toss. Place anchovies as desired on salads. You may also have decanters of olive oil and rice vinegar on the table for individuals to serve themselves in addition. Salt and ground pepper to taste. (Is this as good as it gets? I think so!)

Curried salad Serves 4

1 Tbs. curry powder
2 Tbs. extra-virgin olive oil
1 carrot cut in 1/2-inch dice
1 small onion cut in 1/2-inch dice
1 small tomato seeded and cut in 1/2-inch dice

1 zucchini cut in 1/2-inch dice
1/4 cup dried currants
½ cup canned chickpeas
2 Tbs. fresh lemon juice
Salt and freshly ground pepper to taste

Briefly sauté in olive oil the carrot, onion, tomato, zucchini, currants and chickpeas. In a small bowl, combine the lemon juice, salt and pepper, and 1 Tbs. of olive oil. Pour the contents of the bowl over the salad. Toss until all the ingredients are combined. Season to taste with salt. Serve warm or at room temperature.

Spinach and red cabbage salad Serves 2

5 oz. Packed spinach leaves
8 oz. Grated red cabbage

Wash spinach; discard tough ends and tear large leaves into 2 or 3 pieces. Just before serving, toss spinach with cabbage and dressing (see recipe listed next).

Nobel Prize winning vinaigrette Serves 2 (140/14/0/2-0-2/2-0/0)

2 Tbs. olive oil
2 Tbs. Rice vinegar
2 fresh basil leaves; chopped or 1 Tsp.
dried basil

½ dried tarragon
½ Tsp. Dried mustard
¼ Tsp. Sea salt
Ground pepper to taste

Black bean salad Serves 4

1 cup canned black beans, rinsed and drained
1/2 cup papaya, peeled, seeded and diced
2 Tbs. Red bell pepper, minced
2 Tbs. Green bell pepper, minced

1 scallion, sliced thinly
1 Tsp. Fresh chili, finely chopped
2 Tbs. Fresh lime juice
2 Tsp. Vegetable oil

Combine all ingredients and toss to blend. If desired, chill before serving.

Piquant vegetable salad Serves 4

1 cup cauliflower, chopped

2 cups broccoli, chopped

1 red pepper, chopped

15-ounce can chickpeas, drained and rinsed

3-4 scallions, chopped

2 Tbs. lemon juice

2 Tbs. red wine (or cider) vinegar

1 clove garlic, finely chopped (or 1/8 Tsp. garlic powder)

2 Tsp. Dijon-style mustard

1 Tsp. sugar

If desired, steam cauliflower and broccoli very briefly to blanch. Do not cook completely. Immediately run under cold water to stop cooking process.

Combine cauliflower and broccoli in large bowl with other vegetables. Cover and chill until serving time. In small bowl, stir together lemon juice, vinegar, garlic, mustard, and sugar. Blend thoroughly, cover, and chill until serving time.

Cucumber salad Serves 4

2 cups cucumbers, cut in half lengthwise, seeded and chopped

1 cup sweet red pepper, chopped

1/2 cup carrots, grated or finely diced

1/4 cup scallions or red onion, finely chopped

2 Tsp. fresh ginger, peeled and minced

1 clove garlic, finely chopped

1/2 cup water

1/4 cup white vinegar

Combine all vegetables with ginger, garlic and crushed peppercorns in a medium or large bowl. Add vinegar and mix thoroughly. Cover and refrigerate at least 30 minutes before serving. Best if prepared a day ahead.

SALADS   Meat/Fish/Poultry

Shrimp salad Serves 2 (220/11/24/4-2-2/5-1/173)

2 cups cooked shrimp (8 oz)

2 Tbs. grapeseed or canola oil mayonnaise

2 Tsp. capers

1 stalk celery, chopped

1 Tbs. lemon juice

Freshly ground black pepper

Cut the shrimp into bite-size pieces. Place in a bowl. Add mayonnaise, capers and celery. Sprinkle lemon juice and pepper to taste over the salad. Stir to coat shrimp and blend ingredients. Serve on lettuce leaves.

Salmon salad Serves 2 with ½ cup each (288/21/21/3-2-1/4-3/60)

7.5 oz can of salmon-boneless	Salt and pepper to taste
2 Tbs. grapeseed or canola oil mayonnaise	Optional: 1 Tbs. chopped onion
2 celery stalks, finely chopped	

Mix all ingredients together. May serve with mixed green salad.

Helen of Troy Salad of Tuna Serves 1 (228/11/31/3-2-1/3-1/37)

6 oz can of solid white tuna, drained	1 celery stalk, finely chopped
1 Tbs. grape seed oil mayonnaise	Salt and pepper to taste
½ Tsp. fresh dill or ¼ Tsp. dried dill	Optional: 1 Tbs. chopped onion

Mix all ingredients together. May serve with mixed green salad.

Mexican chicken salad Serves 2

1 cup thinly sliced white daikon	2 Tbs. freshly squeezed lime juice
2 cups (about 8 oz.) diced cooked chicken breast	1 Tsp. salt
1/2 cup thin cucumber slices, halved into crescents	4 cups romaine lettuce, torn in 2-inch pieces
1/4 cup thinly sliced red onion, in crescents	1/4 Tsp. (round) chili powder or 3 to 4 dashes hot pepper sauce
2 Tbs. olive oil	
1/4 cup freshly squeezed orange juice	2 Tbs. coarsely chopped cilantro

Place cut up daikon in a large glass bowl. Add the chicken. Add the cucumber and onion. In a small bowl, whisk together the oil, orange and lime juices, and salt. Mix until blended. If using hot sauce, add it at this point. Pour the dressing over the chicken salad and toss to blend.

Arrange 1 cup of the lettuce on each of four salad plates. Heap a quarter of the chicken salad on each plate. Sprinkle with the chili powder and the cilantro. Serve immediately. This salad is best when freshly made, but it can keep about an hour; after that the citrus flavors fade.

Tamari tuna salad Serves 1 (228/11/31/3-2-1/3-1)

6 oz can of solid white tuna, drained	½ Tsp. Tamari sauce
1 Tbs. Grapeseed or canola oil mayonnaise	Salt and pepper to taste
1 celery stalk, finely chopped	

Mix all ingredients together. May serve with mixed green salad.

Calories / Fat / Protein / Total Carbs-Fiber-Net Carbs / Omega 6-Omega 3 / Cholesterol

Curried chicken salad Serves 2 (206/18/31/5-2-3/4-0)

1 lb. boiled chicken or turkey breast	2 celery stalks- finely chopped
1 Tbs. grapeseed or canola oil mayonnaise	1 Tsp. curry powder
½ Tbs. seasoned rice vinegar	Salt and pepper to taste
1 Tsp. lemon juice	Optional: 1 Tbs. chopped onion

Mix all ingredients together. May serve with mixed green salad.

Call me Ishmael's chicken/turkey salad Serves 2 with ½ cup each (206/18/31/5-2-3/4-0/80)

½ lb. boiled chicken or turkey breast	1 Tsp. lemon juice
1 Tbs. grapeseed or canola oil mayonnaise	2 celery stalks- finely chopped
1 Tbs. organic heavy cream	Salt and pepper to taste
½ Tbs. seasoned rice vinegar	Optional: 1 Tbs. chopped onion

Mix all ingredients together. May serve with mixed green salad.

Vegetarians are giving their life back to the earth by not consuming animals. I agree it would be better if we did not have to kill to live, but the consumption of fish and other meat/poultry promotes greater health through essential oils, proteins and vitamins. I believe we are designed to be omnivores living on healthy oils, green leafy vegetables, fish/poultry/meat as well as nuts, seeds and fruit (in about that order). But for those individuals who prefer to not sacrifice animals, here are some reasonably healthy alternatives.

Brisk lentil and Brussel sprout stew Serves 4

1 cup dried lentils

2 cups Brussel sprouts, quartered

1 carrot, diced

1 cup winter squash, cubed

2 bay leaves

3 cups water

Dash of soy sauce

2 Tsp. brown rice Miso or soy sauce

¼ cup minced fresh parsley

Add first 7 ingredients to a large pot, bring to boil and then reduce heat to low simmer for 30 minutes or until lentils are tender. Remove from heat; add Miso or soy sauce and parsley and serve.

Lentil Dahl Serves 4

1 cup dried lentils

3 cups water

3 peeled tomatoes, diced (11 oz can or fresh) with juice

1 carrot, diced

¼ cup olive oil

1 Tsp. curry powder

½ Tsp. cumin

1 clove garlic, pressed

Salt and pepper to taste

Bring water with lentils to boil, then add tomatoes, carrots, olive oil, curry powder, pressed garlic, salt and pepper. Reduce heat and simmer for 30 minutes or until lentils are tender. Serve with brown rice.

Ratatouille Serves 4   (avoid if you have arthritis? –all "nightshade" vegetables)

1 medium eggplant, diced

2 zucchini cut up

3 peeled tomatoes, diced (fresh or 11 oz can)

6 mushrooms, sliced (fresh or 5-7 oz can)

2 cloves garlic, pressed

1 small onion, sliced

1 Tsp. basil

½ cup olive oil

Salt and pepper to taste

2 fennel seeds (optional)

Sauté eggplant in ½ cup of olive oil. Add zucchini, tomatoes, mushrooms, garlic, onion, basil, water, (and fennel). Bring to boil and simmer for 20-30 minutes on low. Add salt and pepper to taste.

Mexican black bean with wild rice Serves 4

¼ cup olive oil

1 medium onion, chopped

1 green pepper, chopped

6 oz wild rice (dry weight) cooked

½ Tsp. cumin

¼ Tsp. red pepper

1/8 Tsp. coriander

Black beans (15 oz can, drained and rinsed)

3 peeled tomatoes, diced (fresh or 14.5 oz can)

Cook wild rice. Sauté onion, green pepper until tender. Add rice and remaining ingredients and heat thoroughly.

Vegetable jubilee (Pasta primavera without the pasta) Serves 4

10 asparagus spears cut into 1inch pieces

Broccoli flowerets from one head

½ cup snow pea pods

1 yellow squash, sliced

1 zucchini, sliced

5 oz mushrooms, sliced

1 clove garlic, pressed

1/3 cup olive oil

1 Tbs. fresh parsley

1 Tbs. fresh basil

1/3 cup water

6 oz wild rice, cooked

Salt and pepper to taste

Sauté first 7 ingredients for 5 minutes in olive oil, stirring frequently. Add cooked wild rice, parsley, basil, salt, pepper, and water, and heat an additional 2-3 minutes. Serve immediately.

Greek rice pilaf Serves 4

1/3 cup olive oil	½ Tsp. thyme
1 small onion, chopped	¼ Tsp. oregano
1 cup long grain rice	2 cucumbers, diced
2 cups water	1/3 cup crumbled Feta cheese
2 Tsp. brown rice Miso or soy sauce	1 Tbs. diced pimento

Sauté onion and rice in olive oil until brown. Add water, spices, and Miso or soy sauce and bring to boil. Reduce heat and simmer for 15 minutes or until rice is tender and liquid absorbed. Remove from heat and stir in cucumber, Feta cheese and pimento. Serve immediately.

Broccoli quiche (with eggs) Serves 4

Calories 136, Fat 8, Mono 4, Poly 1/1, Sat 2, Carbohydrate 4, Sugar 1, Fiber 2, Protein 12

1 Tbs. olive oil	4 large eggs, lightly beaten
1 cup chopped fresh broccoli	½ cup almond milk
½ cup finely chopped sweet red pepper	½ Tsp. salt
¼ cup finely chopped onion	¼ Tsp. dry mustard
¼ cup water	¼ Tsp. ground red pepper

Combine broccoli, sweet red pepper, onion, and olive oil in a medium saucepan. Cover and cook over medium heat 3 to 5 minutes or until vegetables are crisp-tender. Combine vegetable mixture, beaten eggs and next 5 ingredients in a large bowl, stirring well. Pour mixture into a 9-inch quiche dish coated with olive oil. Bake at 350° for 35 to 40 minutes or until set. Let stand 10 minutes before slicing into wedges.

Dessert

Strawberry smoothie Serves 2 (140/9/6/13-7-6/2-3/0)

1 cup frozen strawberries	½ Tsp. vanilla
15 almonds	(1 pack of Stevia)
1 cup filtered water	

Place the nuts in the blender and blend until chopped into fine pieces. Add the water and blend on high, adding the strawberries one at a time. Blend for 2-3 minutes or until thick. Pour immediately into two bowls and enjoy.

Blueberry smoothie Serves 2 (157/9/6/18-8-10/2-3/0)

1 cup frozen blueberries	½ Tsp. vanilla
15 almonds	(1 pack of Stevia)
1 cup filtered water	

Place nuts in blender and blend until chopped into fine pieces. Add the water and blend on high while adding the blueberries. Blend for 2-3 minutes or until thick. Pour immediately into two bowls and enjoy.

Fresh berries with heavy cream and brandy Serves 2 (116/5/2/15-6-9/0/15)

½ cup fresh blueberries	2 Tbs. organic heavy cream
½ cup fresh raspberries	2 Tsp. Brandy
1 cup fresh strawberries, halved	

Mix berries and distribute evenly into two shallow bowls. Pour 1 Tbs. of cream followed by 1 Tsp. Brandy on fruit.

8 Fresh Strawberries (25/0/1/5-2-3/0/0)

1 Kiwi, sliced (46/0/1/11-3-8/0/0)

Raspberries ½ cup (fresh or frozen) **with 1 Tbs. heavy cream** (88/6/1/9-4-5/0/21)

½ cup Blueberries (fresh or frozen) (42/0/1/10-3-7/0/0)

The *On A Tight Budget* Approach

My suggestion to all who have the option of following the "Money is No Object" approach is to try to incorporate as many of those changes as possible (although it will cost significantly more). Sometimes money is tight but we still want to feel well. I will first present an approach that will greatly improve health without breaking the bank.

The important substitutions are as follows:

- Conventionally grown food instead of *organic, free range, or organic* food
- Peanuts instead of almonds, walnuts, brazil nuts and cashews
- Peanut butter instead of almond butter, cashew butter, tahini
- Frozen vegetables instead of fresh vegetables
- Hamburger and pot roast instead of expensive cuts of meat
- Regular store-bought chicken instead of *free range, organic* chicken
- Chicken thighs and legs instead of chicken breasts
- Cans of tuna instead of fresh wild salmon
- Cans of tuna instead of cans of salmon, kippers or sardines
- The addition of cheese and cottage cheese (unless you have allergies or asthma)- TRY TO AVOID
- Grapes and apples instead of strawberries, blueberries, raspberries, blackberries
- Frozen strawberries and blueberries instead of fresh strawberries and blueberries (I frequently buy frozen fruits and vegetables for convenience)

Important purchases which must be made:

- Light olive oil (the large can), hopefully on sale for about $10. Tastes good (very mild)
- Chromium supplement 200mcg per day (twice that for people with diabetes)
- MSM 3000mg per day (try it to see if it helps joint pains, allergies and energy level)
- Magnesium 250mg and Calcium 500mg with vitamin D, each once or twice daily
- Omega-3 oils (either Cod liver oil: 1 Tbs. per day) or the capsules 2-4 per day

Breakfasts:

2 eggs over-easy cooked in 1Tbs. olive oil, then add 2 Tbs. salsa in the pan and heat.

2 eggs any style with sautéed green pepper and onion

Peanut butter (2 Tbs.) on celery (or spoon)

Leftovers-Chunks of beef from Stew (4 pieces-2 oz)

Italian Sausage (7 oz- 2 sausages) heated in a pan with a little water and olive oil

1/3 cup rolled oats, 1/3-cup oat bran cooked with ¾ cup water for 5 minutes.

1 cup Cottage Cheese with fruit (if no asthma or allergies)

Oat waffles with strawberries (and whipped cream?)

Lunches:

Chicken Salad (½ to 1 cup), 1 oz peanuts

Tuna salad (½ to 1 cup), 1 oz peanuts

Tuna 5 oz can

Sardines 1 can

Leftover chicken, beef or pork with vegetables

Snacks:

Several handfuls of peanuts (1-2 oz of shelled peanuts)
Get the unshelled peanuts; they last longer and are more enjoyable
(Never go anywhere without your peanuts; you may want something healthy to eat)

Turkey Jerky (1-2 oz)

Beef Jerky (1-2 oz)

1-2 ounces of cheese (if no asthma or allergies)

(But **NO** sodas, candy, bagels, donuts, cookies, cakes, popcorn, pretzels, bread, ice cream, water ice)

Suppers:

Pot Roast with vegetables

Chicken Stew with onion and celery

Deep Tuna Pie with French fried onion rings

Beef and Navy Bean Stew

Tuna Salad or Chicken Salad
(Make enough so you can take for lunch)

Chicken with mustard greens

Hamburgers (no bun) with a vegetable

Desserts:

Frozen Strawberry Smoothie

Roasted Cashews (a special occasion)

Oat waffles with strawberries (and whipped cream?)

Fresh fruit or berries (with cottage cheese?)

You have noticed I have eliminated the following foods:
- Pasta, bread, potatoes and rice
- Milk, yogurt, ice cream
- Pizza
- Spaghetti and lasagna
- Philly Cheese Steak Sandwiches (you can eat the inside but not the roll, thank you very much)

Why? Because these foods tend to make you feel tired. Then you don't exercise. Then your waist-hip ratio goes up. Then your risk of diabetes, heart disease, cancer and depression goes up.

So do not worry about your weight. But do worry about your waist.

And you must exercise 13 minutes per day (in the morning). Your heart rate during this 13 minutes must get up to 120-130 beats per minute or more (count your pulse for 10 seconds; it must be 20 or more beats). Exercise bike, climbing stairs, jogging, jumping jacks, aerobics, and swimming, whatever you can do. Just do it.

Recipes for the Tight Budget

Tuna salad Serves 4

2 cans tuna

1 medium onion, grated

4 eggs, hard boiled and chopped

½ cup celery, chopped

1 medium apple, peeled and chopped

½ cup mayonnaise or light olive oil

Salt and pepper to taste

(2 Tbs. pickle relish)

Combine all ingredients, mix well and chill. Be sure to make enough to take for lunch the next day.

Chicken salad Serves 4

1 lb. cooked chicken without bones (boiled or canned)

½ cup celery, chopped

1 medium apple, peeled and chopped

20 red or white grapes

½ cup mayonnaise or light olive oil

1 Tsp. curry powder

1 Tsp. soy sauce

(1 Tsp. lemon juice)

Salt and pepper to taste

Cut up chicken into small cubes. Combine mayonnaise (or olive oil) with curry powder, soy sauce, lemon juice, salt and pepper and stir well. Put all ingredients into a large serving bowl and mix well. Serve chilled.

Deep tuna pie Serves 4

2 large cans of tuna

1 pound green beans, fresh or frozen

1 can cream of mushroom soup

2 Tbs. olive oil

1 can French fried onion rings

Mix tuna and green beans in a casserole dish. Pour the mushroom soup over the tuna and beans. Sprinkle top with onion rings and bake at 450 degrees until top is brown (5-10 minutes).
Save some for lunch the next day. Reheat on stove or in microwave.

Pot roast Serves 4

2 pounds of inexpensive beef, cut into large cubes

4 stalks of celery, cut into 1-inch lengths

2 carrots cut into 1-inch lengths

1 medium onion, sliced

1 small can mushrooms

1 can tomatoes

¼ cup light olive oil

1/8 Tsp. dried basil

Salt and pepper to taste

Heat olive oil in a large pot. Add the beef and onion and sauté until brown. Add remaining ingredients, bring to boil, then reduce heat to low and simmer for 45-60 minutes or until beef is tender. Serve in bowls.

Save some for lunch the next day. Reheat on stove or in microwave.

Beef and navy bean stew Serves 4

2 pounds of inexpensive beef, cut into large cubes

10 oz can of navy beans, rinsed

1 cup water

4 stalks of celery, cut into 1-inch lengths

10 oz package of frozen greens (spinach, collard, turnip, kale, etc.)

1 medium onion, sliced

1/3 cup light olive oil

¼ Tsp. basil

¼ Tsp. curry powder

¼ Tsp. oregano

Heat olive oil in a large pot. Sauté beef. Add remaining ingredients and bring to boil. Reduce heat and simmer on low for 45-60 minutes or until beef is tender.

Save some for lunch the next day. Reheat on stove or in microwave.

Pan-fried chicken w/ vegetables Serves 4

2-3 Lb. Broiler-fryer chicken cut up

3 Tbs. oil (olive or canola)

1/3-cup almonds ground finely into powder

1 Tsp. paprika

1 onion sliced

1 egg

Grind almonds in blender until powdery. Place in a bowl. Beat the egg well in a second bowl. Heat the oil on high in a large heavy skillet. Dip the chicken pieces in the egg, coat with almond flour and place in skillet. Turn frequently to prevent burning for the first 2-3 minutes. Reduce heat to low, cover and let cook for an additional 5 minutes. Turn off heat and let coast for another 10 ten minutes so the chicken will be cooked through but still moist. Serve with steamed broccoli, spinach or other green vegetable to your liking.

Chicken stew Serves 4

2 Lb. Chicken cut up

2 Tbs. oil (olive or canola preferred)

½ cup sliced onion

2-14.5 oz cans diced tomatoes with Italian herbs

½ Lb. frozen zucchini

1 Tsp. dried whole thyme

½ Tsp. fennel seeds, crushed

¼ Tsp. salt

Freshly ground pepper (optional)

Heat oil in a pot over medium-high heat until hot. Add onions and sauté until onion is tender. Add chicken, diced tomatoes with Italian herbs, wine, and zucchini to onion mixture, stirring well to combine. Add thyme, fennel seeds, salt and bring to boil stirring well.

Reduce heat, cover, and simmer 20-25 minutes or until done. Ladle stew into individual bowls, and garnish with freshly ground pepper, if desired.

Tacos and salad Serves 4

1 Lb. ground beef

2 tomatoes sliced into wedges

1-16 oz jar of salsa-mild, medium or hot

Lettuce leaves washed and shredded

6 taco shells

1 onion chopped (optional)

Makings of a green salad

Cook the ground beef and onions in a skillet until brown. Drain the excess juice and then add ½ cup of salsa to the hamburger mixture and stir. Fill the taco shells with the lettuce, hamburger mix, tomato and additional salsa to taste. Enjoy 1-2 tacos as needed. Serve with a tossed green salad.

Bean burritos w/ salad Serves 4

2 cans of refried beans

8 flour tortillas

1-16 oz jar of salsa-mild, medium or hot

Cheddar cheese-grated (if no allergies)

Makings of a green salad

Preheat oven to 350 degrees. Grease a square Pyrex dish with butter or oil. Divide the refried beans among the 8 tortillas and roll the tortillas into tubes. Place in the Pyrex dishes and cover with Salsa (and grated cheese if no allergy symptoms). Bake in oven for 15-20 minutes or until hot inside.

Chinese chicken with broccoli and peanuts Serves 4

2 –3 Lb. Chicken cut up	4 oz. peanuts
1/3 cup oil (olive or canola preferred)	1 Tbs. soy sauce
1 onion sliced	1 Tsp. ginger powder (optional)
1 Lb. broccoli (fresh or frozen)	Salt and pepper to taste

Heat oil in a large heavy skillet. Add chicken and onions. Sauté for 5 minutes or until brown. Add peanuts, soy sauce, ginger powder and salt and pepper, cover and reduce heat. Simmer for 15-20 minutes. Add broccoli and cook additional 5 minutes. May serve with a green salad on the side.

Hey, isn't this just the Atkins' Diet?

What about the low-fat Ornish Diet?

How does this compare to the Protein Power Diet?

9

THE MEDITERRANEAN HUNTER-GATHERER DIET

VERSUS ORNISH, ATKINS AND PROTEIN POWER

1   How Does the Mediterranean Hunter-Gatherer Diet compare to the Diets of Dr. Ornish, Dr. Atkins, and Drs. Eades (Protein Power)?

The following pages include tables comparing these four approaches. The Protein Power plan is very similar to many of the other diets now available. These include the South Beach Diet, the Schwarzbein Principle, Sugar Busters, The Zone, and many others. There are only three very-low carbohydrate diets: the Atkins', Neanderthin, and the Mediterranean Hunter-Gatherer diet (presented in this book). It is clear that we are all trying to present the best information we have in our plans. We continue to learn more each day. The Seven Day Plan (Nutrition for Women: Men, add 50%) that I present is (I believe) the best for improvement of waist circumference, allergies and asthma, inflammatory bowel disease, arthritis, and the prevention of cancer of the colon, breast, prostate and pancreas. This is in addition to all of the benefits ascribed to the Atkins Diet in the ongoing studies at Duke and elsewhere that patients following the Atkins' Diet have greater energy, improved mood, less heartburn, and less pre-menstrual, menstrual, and menopausal problems.

(a)   *The Atkins' Diet*

Dr. Steele always threatens his patients with a quiz when they return to see him. Because healing comes from within, so it just doesn't matter if the doctor knows his stuff. It only matters if the patients know their stuff! So before looking at these tables, you need to take a quiz. It is important that you understand this information, so what better way to find out how much you know than taking a quiz (to prepare you for the test of life).

The Atkins' diet quiz: are you doing the Atkins' diet correctly? Check if you are doing the critical suggestions Dr. Atkins makes in his book but may not repeat in his eating suggestions. See page 186 for the answers.

(1) When to snack? On what do you snack? How much can you have?

(2) What do you want your ratio of omega 6 to omega 3 oils to be? What are the benefits of omega 3 oils? What are good sources of omega 3 oils?

(3) How many grams of fiber should you eat per day? Which supplements are helpful for constipation?

(4) What are possible reactions to dairy products? Which component of dairy promotes allergies? Are butter and heavy cream acceptable to those with allergies?

(5) What about wheat; could keeping the wheat and corn out of your diet be beneficial in the long run?

(6) Is all of that cholesterol and saturated fat bad for you? How does Dr. Atkins suggest you check to see if you are having problems with the diet?

(7) What is metabolic resistance? Is it the same as insulin resistance? What is Syndrome X? How can you tell if you have metabolic resistance? How does that alter your diet?

(8) What is a typical serving size of meat? 4 oz, 6 oz or 8 oz?

(9) Are the calorie requirements of men and women the same? If not, how much more can a typical man eat and still lose weight?

(10) Do you really need to take all of those supplements that Dr. Atkins suggests? Which are the critical supplements; what is the absolute minimum required for success?

(11) What are Lipolysis testing strips? Is this a fancy term for the Ketostix you buy in the pharmacy?

(12) Is ketosis bad for you? We know the induction diet is ketogenic (induces a state of ketosis where you burn fat as fuel instead of carbohydrate). But Dr. Atkins tells you to only be on this diet for the first two weeks. Is the *On-going Weight Loss* diet also ketogenic?

(13) Is ketosis a bad thing? How many grams of carbohydrates are you allowed? Is it 20, 40, or 60 grams and how do you determine this? See page186 for the answer key.

(b) *The Ornish Diet: Is your being a vegetarian the best option for the Earth and you?*

(1) How many calories are included in the typical Ornish day?

(2) Is your being a vegetarian good for the earth?

(3) Is your being a vegetarian good for you?

(4) What is the ratio of omega 6 and omega 3 oils in the Ornish diet?

(5) Is the Ornish program still effective if you do not do the meditation?

(c) *The Protein Power Diet (The diet by Drs. Eades)*

(1) How many calories in the typical Protein Power day?

(2) What is the percentage of calories from protein?

(3) Are there patients who should avoid excess protein?

(4) How many digestible carbohydrates are allowed?

(5) Is this a ketogenic diet?

(6) How much fat and oils do they allow?

Table 9-1

Calories/Fat /Protein/ Total Carbs-Fiber-Net Carbs / Omega 6-Omega 3 / Cholesterol

	Steele Diet for Women (Men may eat 50% more)	Ornish Diet	Atkins Induction Diet
Breakfast	Smoked wild salmon (2 oz.) (130/9/11/0/1-5/30) Eaten with a fork 1 Tbs. Cod liver oil (130/14/0/0/2-8/0) Green tea	Oatmeal ½ cup and 1 Tbs. raisins (181/3/5/27-4-23/0/0) Nonfat yogurt 8 oz (127/0/13/8-0-8/0-0/4) Whole wheat toast 1 slice 60/0/4/10-1-9/0-0/0) 1 Tsp. preserves (18/0/0/4-0-4/0/0) Orange juice 8 oz (112/1/2/26-2-24/0/0)	2 Eggs (140/9/12/2-0-2/3-0/426) 3 Canadian bacon (70/3/11/0/0-0/30) Decaf coffee Atkins' supplements
Lunch	Salmon salad (½ cup) (288/21/21/3-2-1/4-3/62)	Whole wheat burrito with red beans and "dirty rice" (308/3/15/52-13-39/0-0/0) Chutney (27/0/1/8-2-6/0-0/0) Tossed green salad w/ Chopped fresh cilantro (65/0/4/14-4-10/0-0/0)	Cheeseburger 4 oz (378/27/32/0/0-0/91) with 2 strips Bacon (60/5/4/0/0-0/10) No bun Salad w/ dressing (140/7/5/5-2-3/0-0/0) Seltzer
Snack	30 almonds (1 oz) (180/16/7/7-4-3/4-0/0) Green tea	Optional hot beverage	None

	Steele Diet for Women (Men may eat 50% more)	Ornish Diet	Atkins Induction Diet
Dinner	Filet mignon 6 oz (or other lean steak) with sautéed onion (338/27/48/6-2-4/3-0/130) Greens with garlic and olive oil or other fat (140/7/5/5-5-1/0-0/0)	Spinach ravioli (107/1/16/12-2-10/0/3)) Creamed lentil soup with celery (115/1/7/23-6-17/0/0) Garlic croutons (20/0/1/4-0-4/0-0/0) Herb salad (39/0/3/4-2-2/0-0/0)	Shrimp cocktail 4 oz 130/2/23/3-0-3/0-1/173) Clear consommé (20/2/0/0/0-0/0) Rib steak 6 oz (278/20/48/0/0-0/130) Salad w/ dressing 1 Tbs. (140/7/5/5-2-3/0-0/0)
Dessert	Strawberry smoothie (140/9/6/13-7-6/2-3/0)	Vanilla poached fruits (127/0/5/24-4-20/0/0)	Diet Jell-O w/ whipped heavy cream (53/6/0/0/0-0/21)
Calories Fat Protein CHO Fiber Net carbs O-6/O-3 Cholest.	1285 calories 98 gm (882 calories- 68%) 88 gm (352 calories- 28%) 32 gm 20 gm 12 gm (48 calories- 4%) 14 gm/16 gm (1:1) 222 mg	1306 calories 8 gm (72 calories- 6%) 64 gm (256 calories- 20%) 216 gm 40 gm (160 calories- 12%) 176 gm (704 calories- 54%) 0 gm/0 gm 7 mg cholesterol	1409 calories 88 gm (954 calories-57%) 140 gm (648 calories- 39%) 15 gm 4 gm 11 gm (40 calories- 2%) 3 gm/1 gm 881 mg cholesterol

Calories/Fat /Protein/ Total Carbs-Fiber-Net Carbs / Omega 6-Omega 3 / Cholesterol

	Atkins Ongoing Wt Loss	Atkins Maintenance	Protein Power
Breakfast	Western omelet w/ 2 eggs (262/21/14/4-1-3/2-1/556) 3 oz V-8 juice (20/0/0/3-1-2/0-0/0) 2 bran crispbread (24/0/2/8-4-4/0-0/0) Decaf coffee Atkins' supplements	Spinach and cheese omelet (375/30/21/4-1-3/0-0/586) ½ cantaloupe (48/0/1/12-0-12/0-0/0) 4 bran crispbread (48/0/4/16-8-8/0-0/0) Decaf coffee Atkins' supplements	2 Poached eggs on (140/9/12/1-0-1/2-1/426) 1 slice light bread toast w/ 1 Tsp. butter (74/5/2/9-2-7/0-0/10) ½ cup fresh or frozen berries (40/0/1/10-3-7/0-0/0) Coffee, tea or mineral water
Lunch	Chef's salad w/ ham, cheese, chicken and egg (338/19/20/6-4-2/2-1/75) w / oil and vinegar 1 Tbs. (140/14/0/2-0-2/2-0/0) Iced herbal tea	Roast chicken (1 breast) (293/14/38/0-0-0/0-0/111) 8 asparagus stalks w/ lemon (60/0/6/12-4-8/0-0/0) Salad with 2 Tbs. olive oil & vinegar dressing (170/14/2/6-2-4/2-0/0) Club soda	Grilled Chicken Sandwich w/ both buns removed (293/14/38/0-0-0/0-0/111) 1-2 cups of mixed greens, tomato wedges and olives olive oil dressing (170/14/2/6-2-4/2-0/0) ½ cup fresh or frozen berries (40/0/1/10-3-7/0-0/0)
Snack	None	None	1 oz hard cheese 1 peach or ½ Valencia orange (149/8/9/14-3-10/0-0/25)

	Atkins Ongoing Wt Loss	Atkins Maintenance	Protein Power
Dinner	Seafood salad (288/21/21/3-2-1/4-3/30) Poached salmon 312/19/36/2-0-2/3-9/93) Sautéed zucchini with garlic (83/7/2/4-2-2/1-0/0)	French onion soup (210/16/2/15-4-11/0-0/17) Salad w/ dressing (170/14/2/6-2-4/2-0/0) Steamed squash 1 cup (18/0/2/4-2-2/0-0/0) ½ baked potato (72/0/2/17-1-16/0-0/0) w/ 2 Tbs. sour cream (60/5/1/1-0-1/0-0/25) Breaded veal chops 6 oz (360/12/46/10-1-9/0-0/196) 5 oz of dry wine (85/0/0/3-0-3/0-0/0/0)	Grilled or boiled fish (salmon, swordfish, tuna) w/ lemon butter (270/17/27/0/3-9/93) 1 small zucchini, sautéed (83/7/2/4-2-2/1-0/0) 1-2 cups of mixed greens, tomato wedges, carrot curls, radishes and olives w/ olive oil dressing (170/14/2/6-2-4/2-0/0) 4 oz dry white wine
Dessert	½ cup strawberries 25/0/1/6-2-4/0-0/0) in 1 Tbs. heavy cream (53/6/0/0/0-0/21)	Generous cup of fresh fruit (127/0/5/24-4-20/0/0)	Strawberry sorbet (4 frozen strawberries w/ 2 Tbs. heavy cream, pureed until smooth (131/12/1/6-2-4/0-0/42)
Calories Fat Protein CHO Fiber Net carbs O-6/O-3 Chol	1545 calories 100 gm (900 cal- 58%) 94 gm (376 cal- 24%) 38 gm 16 gm 22 gm (88cal- 6%) 20 gm/14 gm 775 mg	2069 calories 105 gm (945 cal- 46%) 132 gm (528 cal- 26%) 130 gm 29 gm 101 gm (404 cal-20%) 4 gm/0 gm 935 mg	1468 calories 100 gm (900 cal- 61%) 97 gm (388 cal- 26%) 66 gm 19 gm 47 gm (188 cal- 13%) 10 gm/10 gm 707 mg

So, looking at…

3. **The Complexity of the Diets**

    (a)   *The Fish Oils: the balance of omega 6 and omega 3 oils*

        (1) The over-consumption of omega 6 oils has been associated with increased numbers of cancers. It is important to try to balance the omega 6 and omega 3 oils in a ratio of close to 2:1.

        (2) The Ornish program, being a very low fat diet, thereby avoids the omega 3 oils in fish. The studies out of Great Britain show a 50% reduction in sudden cardiac death in people consuming an average of 9 grams of omega 3 oils per day[50] (in their kippers, Portuguese sardines and wild North Sea salmon). It appears that the consumption of some of these oils is healthy.

        (3) The Atkins Diet allows but does not encourage the inclusion of these foods. He suggests you take supplements to meet these requirements. In addition to the oils, fish contain many other healthful substances (magnesium, calcium and chromium, as well as many other micronutrients of which we are not even aware) that are also a factor in reducing cardiac death. Eat food rather than supplements.

        (4) Protein Power includes the lemon-flavored Cod liver oil as well as the flax oil (although the flaxseed oil has been associated with possible increase in prostate cancer).

    (b)   *Food Sensitivity: the reduction of foods associated with asthma, allergies, inflammatory bowel disease and arthritis.*

        (1) In many people, milk makes more mucus. And this includes yogurt and low-fat cheeses. It is the protein in milk that promotes the allergic response, not the fat or sugar. The sugar can cause it's own problems with digestion in people who have lactose intolerance.

        (2) Yet Dr. Ornish includes these foods frequently because of the need for some healthy low fat animal protein to supplement the Ornish Diet.

---

[50] Albert CM; Campos H; Stampfer MJ; Ridker PM; Manson JE; Willett WC; Ma J Blood levels of long-chain n-3 fatty acids and the risk of sudden death. *N Engl J Med* 2002 Apr 11;346(15):1113-8.

(3) Dr. Atkins mentions the possibility of food intolerance but has cheese included in many of his suggestions to add fat without adding excess protein.

(4) Dr. Atkins reintroduces a high fiber wheat product in his OWL diet to increase fiber and reduce constipation. This is further increased in his maintenance diet. There is good evidence that many of us do not tolerate wheat and feel better when we avoid it entirely.

(5) There is some evidence (from studies in the 1960's) that the nightshade vegetables (tomatoes, eggplant, potatoes and peppers) may be associated with arthritis in some people.[51] I try to give people the option of trying to avoid these foods to see if there is any difference.

(c) *The Ketogenic Diet: the maintenance of mild ketosis and the attendant antioxidant state.*

(1) Work done by Cahill and others suggests that the ketogenic diet reduces oxidative stress and aging.

(2) Many people eating a ketogenic diet consume fewer calories. It is well shown that calorie restriction increases longevity in all animals tested.

(3) A lower glycemic diet also reduces many of the promoters of aging, including insulin levels and the glycation of proteins (see chapter 2 and 3). There is no food lower in glycemic index than fat.

(4) All heart disease risk parameters improve in patients on the ketogenic diet.

(5) All parameters of diabetes control improve on the ketogenic diet.

(d) *The Glycemic Index*

(1) Dr. Ornish writes about the glycemic index and the importance of avoiding simple sugars and starch in his book <u>Eat More and Weigh Less</u>, but the glycemic index of his diet is high. Sugar is sugar, be it from fruit or cane sugar or chutney or milk. The high starch content of his diet in the form of rice, beans, tortillas, and oatmeal will also raise blood sugar and insulin levels.

---

[51] Panush RS. Possible role of food sensitivity in arthritis. A*nn Allergy* 1988 Dec;61(6 Pt 2):31-5.

(2) The other three diets are very low glycemic, except when Dr. Atkins begins to add back potatoes and bread in his maintenance diet.

(e) ***The Cholesterol Content***

(1) The cholesterol content of the Ornish diet is extremely low, as is the fat content. But the evidence that cholesterol is bad for us is lacking except perhaps in patients with genetically high cholesterol levels (about 5% of us) or those with poorly controlled diabetes. Those patients should avoid shrimp, lobster, and egg yolks as well as excess butter and cream.

(2) All of the other diets have similar cholesterol contents (all less than 1 gram per day). One gram is 1/30 of one ounce and has the total caloric content of nine calories (less than 1/2 of 1 percent of the total calories of any of the weight loss diets). Therefore, do not worry. But to be prudent, have your health care practitioner check your cholesterol, LDL, HDL and Triglyceride levels no matter which diet you choose.

4. The Answers to the Quizzes

(a) *Atkins' Diet Quiz*

When to snack? On what do you snack? How much can you have?
> According to the Atkins program, you will not need to snack.

What do you want your ratio of omega 6 to omega 3 oils to be? What are the benefits of omega 3 oils? What are good sources of omega 3 oils?
> Although Atkins suggested you eat fish, he never suggested how much fish to eat. But he did suggest you take his vitamin pack.

How many grams of fiber should you eat per day? Which supplements are helpful for constipation?
> Dr. Atkins admitted his diet was low in fiber so he suggested patients with constipation take fiber supplements (many of my patients complain of too frequent bowel movements if any problem at all). The exception to this is older patients who do not consume adequate fluids due to urinary leakage or prostate problems.

What are possible reactions to dairy products? Which component of dairy promotes allergies? Are butter and heavy cream acceptable to those with allergies?

Dr. Atkins does suggest that people may have an adverse reaction to dairy, but he did little to address how to substitute for the cheese and other high-protein dairy in his diet plan.

What about wheat; could keeping the wheat and corn out of your diet be beneficial in the long run?

In his maintenance diet, Dr. Atkins adds back wheat fiber to add fiber to his diet, all the while admitting many people do not tolerate wheat well.

Is all of that cholesterol and saturated fat bad for you? How does Dr. Atkins suggest you check to see if you are having problems with the diet?

About 5% of the population (people with genetically high cholesterol) will have significant problems with the amount of saturated fat and cholesterol in the Atkins plan. In addition, people with diabetes will initially have elevations of their cholesterol levels on the high fat diet, which will return to normal as their diabetes goes away. Most physicians will treat these patients with cholesterol lowering drugs until the diabetes resolves.

What is metabolic resistance? Is it the same as insulin resistance? What is Syndrome X? How can you tell if you have metabolic resistance? How does that alter your diet?

Yes, they are the same. If your waist is over 35 inches, you probably have insulin resistance (metabolic resistance). Avoid simple carbohydrates (sugar, starches and sweet fruits) and greatly increase your intake of healthy fats.

What is a typical serving size of meat? 4 oz, 6 oz or 8 oz?

Dr. Atkins never made this clear, which is part of the reason that many women never lost weight on the Atkins' Diet. The size of your palm is 4 oz. This is the typical serving for women for lunch. Six ounces is a good amount for dinner. Men can eat 50% more for each meal (i.e. 6 oz. for lunch and 9 oz. for dinner).

Are the calorie requirements of men and women the same? If not, how much more can a typical man eat and still lose weight?

Women need to consume about 1200 calories to lose weight, while men can eat 1800 calories per day (so who said life was fair?). So women need to eat less to succeed, while most men can eat more. If you exercise to excess, you can eat more (2-3 hours per day).

Do you really need to take all of those supplements that Dr. Atkins suggests? Which are the critical supplements; what is the absolute minimum required for success?

The most important supplements are discussed in Chapter 10 on supplements. If you follow those recommendations you will save a lot of money and still stay healthy.

What are Lipolysis testing strips? Is this a fancy term for the Ketostix you buy in the pharmacy?

Yes. I encourage you to check for ketosis, because if you fall out of ketosis you are cheating with too many carbs!

Is ketosis bad for you? We know the induction diet is ketogenic (induces a state of ketosis where you burn fat as fuel instead of carbohydrate). But Dr. Atkins tells you to only be on this diet for the first two weeks. Is the On-going Weight Loss diet also ketogenic?

Ketosis appears to reduce markers of aging and maintain health. I encourage my patients to maintain ketosis to reduce aging. Alternate day feeding of rats keeps them young (physically and sexually) so they survive twice as long and have twice as much fun!

Is ketosis a bad thing? How many grams of Net Carbs are you allowed? Is it 20, 40, or 60 grams and how do you determine this?

The Ketostix are key to determining how many carbs you may consume. If you fall out of ketosis, fall back and reduce your carbs.

(b) ***The Ornish Diet***: *Is your being a vegetarian the best option for the Earth and you?*

How many calories are included in the typical Ornish day?

This varies between 900 and 1200 calories per day for men and women.

Is your being a vegetarian good for the earth?

If you believe that killing animals for humans to survive is wrong, then being a vegetarian is good. But much of the animal kingdom has no qualms to feeding their offspring meat. We are probably meant to be omnivores, consuming all foods present in the wild state of nature (not what you might find at your local fast food restaurant).

Is your being a vegetarian good for you?

The simple answer is no. We need vitamin B-12 (only present in the flesh of animals). We need omega-3 oils in fish for our brains and heart (albeit also present in flaxseed). We need healthy protein without the high levels of simple starches in beans, rice and whole grains.

What is the ratio of omega 6 and omega 3 oils in the Ornish diet?

> Since fish is eliminated from the diet, there is very little omega 3 oils in this diet.

Is the Ornish program still effective if you do not do the meditation?

> The unpublished data suggests that people who do not do the meditation component of the program do not benefit from reduced cardiovascular risks.

(c) *The Protein Power Diet*

How many calories in the typical Protein Power day?

> Around 1500 calories per day (although again a difference is not made between the sexes). Men require about 50% more calories than women do, while women require fewer calories than men to have the same weight loss and health outcomes.

What is the percentage of calories from protein?

> Despite the title of their book, this is not a high-protein diet but a high fat diet. But this is actually healthy as has been discussed above.

Are there patients who should avoid excess protein?

> All patients with significant kidney or liver disease are recommended to avoid excess protein. But excess fat appears to be safe as long as your cholesterol is monitored and you do not cheat with sugar.

How many digestible carbohydrates are allowed?

> The Protein Power diet allows well over 40-50 grams of digestible carbohydrates per day.

Is this a ketogenic diet?

> No. If we consume more than 30-40 grams of carbohydrates per day, most of us will not be in ketosis. And since there is good evidence that ketosis may reduce oxidative stress and aging, it may be reasonable to reduce this amount down to 20-30 grams per day.

How much fat and oils do they allow?

> Their sample day includes 61% of their calories from fat. This diet will curb your appetite and lower your insulin resistance as has been seen in many patients. My suggestion is still to consider the Mediterranean Hunter-Gatherer diet to see if you can claim even greater health.

A Balanced Diet is the Foundation of Health

Get Most of Your Nutrients from Good Food

10

NUTRITIONAL SUPPLEMENTS

First and foremost, nutritional supplements will not necessarily prevent a disease from developing in a specific patient. You can take Vitamin E, selenium and eat more broccoli than is humanly possible and still develop prostate cancer (I have seen it happen). But overall the taking of certain supplements is associated with a lower risk of certain diseases (see references in sections below):

- Chromium (inadequate in our soil and food): appears to reduce heart disease, diabetes and depression.
- Selenium: adequate intake is associated with much less prostate, colorectal and lung cancer (Brazil nuts are an excellent source).

1   Why Take Supplements?

Much of our food is grown in depleted soil with the help of nitrogen fertilizers- more bushels per acre but nothing in it- at least not much of the micronutrients we need. Eating organic is important for our bodies as well as the environment. This is why it is important to grow as much of your own food as possible and eat it fresh and raw. The following supplements can hedge your bets and ensure some semblance of complete nutrition although if you could grow all of your food (in the South of France) you would probably not need to take supplements.

2   The Top Three Supplements

There are three supplements, however, that actually make people feel (and look) better. I never miss taking these three. If I am out of town and my cod liver oil is in the refrigerator at home, I will make sure to eat salmon or sardines every day. See the following pages for doses and further information.

(a) *Chromium (reduces insulin resistance)*

Chromium is helpful in diabetes, depression, and to maintain lean body mass. I have found it very effective for improving mood although some patients have found it may give them too much energy. When older rodents are given chromium they behave like younger rodents.[52] Oh, to be a younger rodent.... The daily dose of chromium polynicotinate is 200 mcg each morning. Recent studies suggest possible harm from the picolinate form of the supplement. No suggestion of harm has been seen from the polynicotinate form, which is what is now recommended.

(b) *Omega-3 oils in cod liver oil (stabilizes electrical membranes)*

The consumption of omega-3 oils is associated with a 50% reduction in sudden cardiac death[53] as well as improvement of depression, ADD, schizophrenia and bipolar disorder.[54] It allows me to be nice to my wife. Try it, husbands (and wives?). If you won't eat the salmon or sardines, try the cod liver oil. The amount is 2-3 ounces of fatty fish or 1 Tbs. of cod liver oil (unfortunately this is 6-9 capsules of the fish oil).

(c) *MSM (methylsulfonylmethane- an important sulfur source for healthy connective tissues)*

MSM is present in rainwater and all living things (but not in dead things like most of our food). MSM has been shown effective in knee arthritis and allergic rhinitis. Patent applications suggest it is helpful for tendonitis, asthma, acne, snoring and wrinkles. This supplement makes your knees feel normal and the rest of you feel like you are16 years old (which occasionally gets me in trouble with my wife- that's why I take the Omega-3 oils). The dose is 3-4,000 mg in the morning (or 1 Tsp. of the MSM powder mixed in water).

3   Safety and Efficacy of the Three Key Nutritional Supplements

(a) *Chromium polynicotinate* (200-400mcg daily; twice daily in diabetes)

In the belief that an elevated insulin level promotes aging and disease, chromium is the supplement for you. Chromium is not in our food in adequate amounts so deficiency is common, particularly in patients with diabetes or pre-diabetes.

---

[52] McCarty MF. Longevity effect of chromium pioclinate-'rejuvenation' of hypothalamic function? *Med Hypotheses* 1994 Oct;43(4):253-65.

[53] Albert CM; Campos H; Stampfer MJ; Ridker PM; Manson JE; Willett WC; Ma J Blood levels of long-chain n-3 fatty acids and the risk of sudden death. *N Engl J Med* 2002 Apr 11;346(15):1113-8.

[54] Nemets B; Stahl Z; Belmaker RH Addition of omega-3 fatty acid to maintenance medication treatment for recurrent unipolar depressive disorder. *Am J Psychiatry* 2002 Mar;159(3):477-9.

(1) Improves Diabetes and Insulin Resistance

Greatly improves blood sugars in patients with Type 2 diabetes. Supplemental Chromium improved the blood glucose, insulin, cholesterol, and hemoglobin A1C in people with Type 2 diabetes in a dose dependent manner. (Dose was 500 mcg twice daily) Follow-up studies have confirmed these studies.[55]

Patients with diabetes require more chromium. Urine losses of chromium over many years may exacerbate an already compromised chromium status in patients with type 2 diabetes and might contribute to the developing insulin resistance seen in patients with type 2 diabetes. Patients with type 2 diabetes had mean levels of plasma chromium around 33% lower and urine values almost 100% higher than those found in healthy people.[56]

Improves Gestational Diabetes: Daily intake of 8 mcg/kg body weight was more effective than 4 mcg/kg in women with gestational diabetes. The mechanism of action of chromium involves increased insulin binding, increased insulin receptor number, and increased insulin receptor activity.[57]

Markedly reduces steroid-induced diabetes: diabetes medications were reduced by 50% in patients on steroids treated with chromium 600 mcg per day.[58]

Chromium effective in Type 1 diabetes: 28-year-old woman with an 18-year history of type 1 diabetes mellitus whose Hgb A1c (the test for diabetes control: normal is up to 6.1%) declined from 11.3% to 7.9% 3 months after initiation of chromium, 200 micrograms 3 times daily.[59]

(2) Improves Chronic Depression

In patients with symptoms of chronic depression, chromium supplementation led to remission of dysthymic symptoms.[60]

(3) Improves Heart Disease

Reduces cardiac disease in a population genetically predisposed to insulin resistance.[61]

---

[55] Anderson RA, J Am Coll Nutr 1998 Dec;17(6):548-55 Chromimum, glucose intolerance and diabetes.

[56] Morris BN et al, J Trace Elem Med Biol 1999 Jul;13(1-2):57-61. Chromium homeostasis in patients with type II (NIDDM) diabetes.

[57] Anderson RA, J Am Coll Nutr 1998 Dec;17(6):548-55 Chromimum, glucose intolerance and diabetes.

[58] Ravina A et al. Diabet Med 1999 Feb:16(2):164-7 Reversal of corticosteroid-induced diabetes mellitus with supplemental chromium.

[59]Fox GN, Sabovic C, J Fam Pract 1998 Jan;46(1):83-6 Chromium picolinate supplementation for diabetes mellitus.

[66] McLeod MN, Gaynes BN, Golden RN. Chromium potentiation of antidepressant pharmacotherapy for dysthymic disorder in 5 patients. *Clin Psychiatry* 1999 Apr;60(4):237-40.

(4) No evidence of toxicity in doses of 500 mcg twice daily

No evidence of toxicity in rats at 100mg/kg for six months: Rodents feed chromium picolinate 100 mg/kg for six months (several thousand times the upper limit of the estimated safe dose) showed no toxic effects of chromium on liver or kidney. This was documented by histologic examination (the equivalent of an autopsy with microscopic evaluation of organs).[62]

Toxicity has not been reported in clinical studies. A study showing DNA breaks with picolinate has been severely criticized (similar to pouring LSD on cell cultures and seeing DNA breaks).[63]

One case of renal insufficiency has been reported with chromium picolinate overdose: A case of kidney failure thought to be possibly secondary to chromium picolinate (2500 mcg per day for 3 months). One year later, all laboratory values were within normal limits.[64]

(5) Does chromium make you think and feel younger?

Supplementation of chromium in rodents appears to fool the hypothalamus (the part of the brain that controls sexual hormone production and release) into behaving younger; the hormones and behavior of the chromium-supplemented rodents were similar to much younger rodents.[65]

(b)   *Omega-3 oils in fatty fish and cod liver oil* (1 Tbs. of cod liver oil daily)

(1) How to get the Omega-3 oils into your diet

One Tablespoon of cod liver oil provides the 9 grams of Omega-3 oils, which is equivalent to the dosage used in most studies. Be sure to keep these oils in the refrigerator or they will turn rancid (and smell fishy- and oxidized oils are harmful). I previously recommended Flax oil and Flaxseed but these have recently been suspected of possibly increasing prostate cancer. The cod liver oil provides the same omega-3 oils and has not been associated with problems. The cod liver oil does have a lot of vitamin D, so I would avoid extra vitamin D in the calcium supplement and multivitamin.

---

[61] Mahdi GS. *Lancet* 1995 Apr;345:982-2. Coronary risk factors in people from the Indian subcontinent.
[62] Anderson RA, Bryden NA, Polansky MM. Lack of toxicity of chromium picolinate in rats. *J Am Coll Nutr* 1997 Jun;16(3):273-9.
[63] Speetiens JK et al. The nutritional supplement chromium picolinate cleaves DNA. *Chem Res Toxicol* 1999 Jun;12(6):483-7.
[64] Cerulli J et al. Chromium picolinate toxicity. Ann Pharmacother 1998 Apr;32(4):428-31 .
[65] McCarty MF. Longevity effect of chromium picolinate-'rejuvenation' of hypothalamic function? Med Hypothese 1994 Oct;43(4):253-65.

Eating a total of 12 ounces per week of salmon, kipper herring or sardines will also provide an average of 9 grams per day. I try to eat sardines for lunch several days per week. I particularly like the Bristling Sardines in 2 layers packed in olive oil by Crown Prince. Avoid the farm-raised salmon because they have much less of the Omega-3 oils (because they are fed "dog food" and often given antibiotics to prevent disease). Even the organic food stores carry farm-raised salmon so try to find either the wild Alaskan salmon or wild North Sea or Norwegian salmon.

If you do not want to take a tablespoon of the oil, the oil may be used in an oil and rice vinegar dressing (make fresh or keep refrigerated as cod liver oil will go rancid if heated or left at room temperature). Try to avoid the capsules of flax oil or fish oils. First, the dose is 9 capsules per day (too much and too expensive). In addition, these capsules frequently contain rancid oils, so I would try to stick with the fresh bottles of oils or the actual fish themselves- sardines are the perfect food).

(2) Reduces extra beats or skipped beats of the heart

Consuming an average of 9 grams per day has been associated with a 50% reduction of sudden cardiac death in 2 British trials (this was shown using the fatty fish listed above, which also contain magnesium which can itself reduce cardiac arrhythmias). For this reason the omega-3 oils can be very helpful in people with extra beats or skipped beats of the heart, particularly if taken in conjunction with magnesium.

(3) Improves mood disorders and thought disorders

The psychiatrists are very excited about the improvements they are seeing in patients with depression, schizophrenia, bipolar disorder and attention deficit disorder using the capsules of fish oils. Again, I would try to eat fish or use the fresh oils and avoid the capsules.

(4) Can act as an anticoagulant

The supplementation of omega-3 oils should be stopped about a week before any major surgery. The same goes for Vitamin E, aspirin, as well as gingko, garlic, ginger or ginseng (the four G's).

(5) What is the ideal balance of Omega-3 and Omega –6 oils?

From my reading the ratio of omega-3 to omega-6 should be from one to two up to one to four. The present average in this country is between one to ten up to one to fifty if you only consume processed foods. The Mediterranean Hunter-Gatherer diet has a ratio between one to two up to one to four depending on how much fatty fish you eat.

(6) Should we supplement with gamma linoleic acid (GLA) as well?

Most of us can convert linoleic acid omega-6 oil in our bodies and our diets) to GLA. With illness and aging some of this ability is lost. GLA has been shown to improve eczema, neurologic complications of diabetes, breast pain and premenstrual syndrome. The dose of Evening Primrose oil from the studies is 3-6 grams per day.

The problem I see is that most of us already consume too many omega-6 oils in our diets. Some animal data suggests that omega-6 oils promote the growth of cancer cells. There is 7 times the amount of LA as GLA in Evening Primrose oil. It probably makes sense for most of us to allow our bodies to produce our own GLA (we naturally produce 100 to 1000mg per day by some estimates).

(c)   *MSM (methylsulfonylmethane) (3,000-4,000 mg in the morning)*

When our ancestor Eve was in equatorial Africa and she became hungry, she wouldn't run to the Acme Grocery Store or the Seven Eleven for something to eat. She would go out into her yard (she had a really big yard) and find something to eat, still living, either on a bush or tree or perhaps running along. And she would eat it raw. What is interesting about this is that there are nutrients that are in fresh foods (still on the plant) but not in the best organic foods at the organic food stores. An example of these nutrients is methylsulfonylmethane or MSM.

(1) The Importance of Sulfur in Metabolism

MSM is present in fresh fruits and vegetables (still on the plant or just picked minutes ago), but degrades rapidly during storage or with heating or processing. Also present in raw fish and meat (and rare beef and other meat) and in rainwater. It appears to be an important intermediary in the natural global sulfur cycle.[66] It is the non-toxic, non-odor producing metabolite of DMSO (dimethylsulfoxide, the breakdown product of rotting trees that is part of the Earth's sulfur cycle; DMSO acts as an excellent natural source of sulfur for plants and animals). MSM has been shown to be present in the milk and urine of humans and other animals.

The amount of MSM ingested is one of the rate-limiting steps for methionine synthesis, an important sulfur containing amino acid in the creation of healthy connective tissue and the control of inflammation. This nutrient is important in creating healthy connective tissue (contributes to the body's production of chondroitin sulfate that forms the cartilage in our joints) and controlling inflammation of allergies, arthritis, and tendonitis.

---

[66] Richmond VL. Incorporation of methylsulfonylmethane sulfur into guinea pig serum proteins. *Life Sciences* 1989 Jul; 39(3):263-8.

Methionine deficiency (from the lack of good sulfur sources in our diets such as raw egg yolk) can lead to degenerative diseases. These diseases include arthritis, allergies and asthma, cancer, insomnia, muscle cramps, tendonitis, and depressed mood. It is estimated that 40% of the elderly have severe sulfur deficiency, which leads to many of their problems in aging.

MSM is a precursor for S-adenosyl-L-methionene (SAMe), which has been shown to be effective for arthritis and depression (but SAMe is much more expensive). MSM has been shown to be helpful in patients with interstitial cystitis and the urethral syndrome.[67] It also reportedly reduces wrinkles and promotes healthy nails and hair. Acne and constipation are also improved, although some patients report loose stool at times with the use of MSM.

(2) What is the correct dose of MSM?

The duration of action of MSM (the half-life in the blood) has been calculated to be 38 hours in the Rhesus monkey.[68] It appears the intestinal bacteria may be responsible for some of the incorporation of MSM into essential sulfur amino acids such as methionine.

Methylsulfonylmethane (MSM) 3000mg once in the morning is the dose used in the knee arthritis study and the allergic rhinitis study. (Buy the 1000mg tablets or capsules, or I buy the powder and take 1 Tsp. each morning, which equals 4 grams of MSM. The powder is, however, a little bitter). The major side effect of therapy in these studies was loose stool.

4   Mineral Supplements

(a)   *Magnesium* (250mg once or twice daily)

Maintains the health of bone by facilitating the absorption and metabolism of calcium. In fact, if you take calcium without magnesium you can develop a relative magnesium deficiency and worsening osteoporosis.

Prevents constipation by maintaining adequate magnesium levels. Helps lower blood pressure in patients with hypertension. Reduces cardiac arrhythmias (extra beats of the heart) in patients with palpitations or heart disease. Helps reduce sudden death in patients with dilated hearts and congestive heart failure.

---

[67] Layman DL, Jacob SW. The absorption, metabolism and excretion of dimethyl sulfoxide by rhesus monkeys. *Life Sci* 1985 Dec;37(25):2431-7.

(b)   *Calcium* (250-500mg once or twice daily)

Calcium is required for bone health and the prevention osteoporosis. The correct ratio of calcium to magnesium is between 2:1 and 1:1. This means if you are taking 1,000mg of calcium, you need to take at least 500mg of magnesium. It makes sense to take calcium with added Vitamin D (total of 800 units per day) because most of us do not get adequate sun exposure for adequate Vitamin D conversion.

5   Possibly Useful Supplements: The Antioxidants

Antioxidants protect our mitochondria (the part of the cell that produces energy to run and repair our cells) and help keep the mitochondria producing enough energy so the cell can continue to repair itself and thereby remain healthy. Antioxidants also help reduce the super-oxide radicals that produce cell damage, aging and cancer.

Most of the studies showing an association of antioxidants with improved health outcomes have been looking at foods rich in the vitamin E (mostly nuts and oils) and vitamin K (green leafy vegetables). Eating good food also helps our bodies produce alpha lipoic acid and coenzyme Q-10 (the ketogenic diet has been associated with improved oxidative state, less oxidative stress and improved coenzyme Q-10 function. It therefore may not be essential that we supplement with these.

The one supplement from this group that is important to all of us is selenium. Most of us do not get adequate selenium from our diets because the best sources of selenium are Brazil nuts and other foods grown in selenium rich soil (Brazil and North Dakota).

(a)   *Selenium* (200mcg once daily)

If you live in North Dakota or Brazil you get sufficient selenium in your diet and water to promote good health. The rest of us are probably not getting enough. Taking a supplement of 200 mcg was associated with 63% fewer prostate cancers, 56% fewer colorectal cancers, and 47% fewer lung cancer in average follow-up of 4 ½ years in a recent study. The British Medical Journal suggested that taking selenium was more effective than stopping smoking in reducing lung cancer. Ex-smokers have ongoing inflammation due to the tars and other irritants already present. The antioxidant effect of selenium (and vitamin E?) appears to protect the lung from these tars.

Selenium supplementation has been shown safe in doses of 100-200 mcg per day (3 Brazil nuts). Selenium can be toxic over 800 mcg per day (nausea and stomach distress). People who eat a significant amount of fish may only need this supplements 2-3 times per week (the ocean still has adequate selenium; just do not eat the farm-raised fish). I eat 3-6 Brazil nuts per day and lots of fish.

(b) *Alpha Lipoic Acid* **(300mg once daily; twice daily if neurologic disorders)**

Alpha Lipoic Acid is an antioxidant that prevents or improves nerve damage caused by diabetes. The dose from the studies for diabetes is 300 mg twice daily.[69] Supplementation with alpha-lipoic acid can improve insulin sensitivity in patients with type-2 diabetes.[70] It also decreases oxidative stress even in diabetic patients with poor sugar control and kidneys that are already leaking protein.[71] Patients with diabetes, nerve damage or dementia may want to try the 250-300mg twice daily for 6-8 weeks to see if there is improvement in their condition.

(c) *CoEnzyme Q-10* **(100mg daily; three times daily if neurologic disorders)**

Reduces mitochondrial gene deletion, which is associated with heart failure, memory loss, and diabetes. There have been a few studies suggestive that supplementing with coenzyme Q-10 may reduce heart failure and the recurrence of breast cancer. It also appears to be very effective for neurodegenerative diseases such as Parkinson's disease, Huntington's Chorea and Alzheimer's disease. The dose for treatment is 100mg three times daily, although doses up to 600mg twice daily has been used in Parkinson's with excellent results. It has also been shown to reduce periodontal disease (the major cause of the loss of teeth).

(d) *Vitamin K*

(1) Osteoporosis, Atherosclerosis, and Alzheimer's

Vitamin K is critical not only in blood clotting, but now it is recognized as a critical component in maintaining the health of our bones, blood vessels and brain. Most people are not eating the necessary amount of vitamin K. The best sources of vitamin K are the dark green leafy vegetables (broccoli, spinach, kale, red leaf lettuce, etc), but these require the conversion of vitamin K-1 to K-2 by the bacteria in our intestine.

(2) Vitamin K Content in Foods

The highest concentrations (3000-6000 micrograms/kg) are found in dark-green leafy vegetables and herbs, such as kale, parsley, collard greens, mustard greens, turnip greens, spinach and green cabbage. Intermediate concentrations (1000-2000 micrograms/kg) are found in plants with paler leaves such as white cabbage and lettuce or in green, non-leafy vegetables such as broccoli and Brussel sprouts.

---

[69] Ruhnau KJ et al. Effects of 3-week oral treatment with the antioxidant thioctic acid (alpha-lipoic acid) in symptomatic diabetic polyneuropathy. *Diabet Med* 1999 Dec;16(12):1040-3.

[70] Jacob S et al. Oral administration of RAC-alpha-lipoic acid modulates insulin sensitivity in patients with type-2 diabetes mellitus: a placebo-controlled pilot trial. *Free Radic Biol Med* 1999 Aug;27(3-4):309-14.

[71] Borcea V et al. *Free Radic Biol Med* 1999 Jun;26(11-12):1495-500.

Other foods such as dairy products, meat dishes and cereal-based foods (bread, biscuits, cakes, desserts etc.), although not in themselves particularly rich in vitamin K1 (< 200 micrograms/kg), may contribute significantly to intakes when consumption of green vegetables is poor.

Fats and oils contain variable amounts of vitamin K1 with the highest concentrations (300-1300 micrograms/kg) in canola and olive oils. Vitamin K requires oil to be absorbed (fat-soluble). Hence the need for oil on your salad and vegetables. Low fat diets, Olestra, bile acid binders, and mineral oil laxatives reduce absorption of vitamin K (and other fat-soluble nutrients).

(3) Other Interesting Effects of Vitamin K

Vitamin K also has been shown to inhibit IL-6 (Interleukin-6, a mediator of inflammation (Ferrucci L) (Weber P)). Patients with apolipoprotein E-4 (inherited abnormality that is associated with Alzheimer's) clear Vitamin K more rapidly and also have osteoporosis. It is postulated the abnormal calcium metabolism may also be damaging the brain (Kohlmeier M).

Vitamin K prevented atherosclerosis in rabbits bred to have high cholesterol levels (Kawashima H). Some improvement seen in animals with diabetes with vitamin K supplementation. Vitamin K does not cause increased blood clotting, even at doses of 250mg/kg in laboratory animals (Ronden J). Warfarin has been shown in one large study to be associated with increased fracture rate in older women (another showed no effect) (Booth S). There is a blood test available for undercarboxylated osteocalcin, which predicts risk of fracture in institutionalized women (aged 70-97 years), odds ratio of 3.1 for an elevated level at baseline and followed for 3 years (Szulc P).

(4) Our intake of Vitamin K is too low

Undercarboxylation (lack of vitamin K effect) of the matrix GLA proteins (MGP) in your blood vessel walls is a risk factor for vascular calcification and that the present RDA values are too low to ensure full carboxylation of MGP.[72] A substantial part of the population is mildly deficient in vitamin K, and at later ages this deficiency may contribute to increased bone fracture risk, arterial calcification, and cardiovascular disease.[73] Strenuous exercise may result in hypoestrogenism and amenorrhoea. As a consequence a low peak bone mass and rapid bone loss are often seen in relatively young athletes. All participants received vitamin K supplementation (10 mg/day). In the low-estrogen group vitamin K supplementation induced a

---

[72] Schurgers LJ, Dissel PE, Spronk HM, Soute BA, Dhore CR, Cleutjens JP, Vermeer C. Role of vitamin K and vitamin K-dependent proteins in vascular calcification. *Kardiol* 2001;90Phytonadione:57-63.

[73] Vermeer C, Schurgers LJ. A comprehensive review of vitamin K and vitamin K antagonists. *Hematol Oncol Clin North Am* 2000 Apr;14(2):339-353.

15-20% increase of bone formation markers and a parallel 20-25% decrease of bone resorption markers. This shift is suggestive for an improved balance between bone formation and resorption.[74]

(5) Recommended doses of Vitamin K

Five to six servings of serious green leafy vegetables per day (Kale, Swiss chard, collards, spinach, dandelion greens, green and red cabbage, broccoli, red and green leaf lettuce, romaine lettuce, endive, Chinese cabbage, bok choy, fennel, celery, cucumbers, cauliflower, zucchini, Brussel sprouts).

The recommended dose is 10mg per day of Vitamin K-1 for people at risk for Vitamin K deficiency, atherosclerosis, osteoporosis, and Alzheimer's disease (not the 100mcg dose).

(e)   *Vitamin E* (Eat almonds; avoid supplements unless for macular degeneration)

Again, most of the data for the benefits of vitamin E come from nutritional studies linking a diet rich in vitamin E (from oils and nuts) to lower rates of disease, in particular lung and prostate cancer, heart disease and Alzheimer's disease. Many of the studies of vitamin E supplementation have been disappointing so my recommendation is to increase your intake of healthy oils (olive and nut oils) and nuts. Two recent studies suggested that supplemental vitamin E may actually increase heart disease.

The one area of research that may be promising is Alzheimer's disease. Large doses of vitamin E (2,000 IU per day) did show slight slowing of progression of memory loss in patients with Alzheimer's disease (but not enough to be clinically important). A study also showed a 40% reduction of prostate cancer in smoking Scandinavian men, but most of us do not smoke nor are we from Scandinavia.

If you would like to take a supplement, 200-400 IU is enough for most of us. The correct formulation is natural vitamin E (known as d-alpha tocopherol plus mixed tocopherols). May increase risk of bleeding if taken with aspirin. Stop one week prior to surgery. My suggestion is to eat nuts and healthy oils to get your vitamin E.

---

[74] Craciun AM, Wolf J, Knapen MH, Brouns F, Vermeer C. Improved bone metabolism in female elite athletes after vitamin K supplementation. *Int J Sports Med* 1998 Oct;19(7):479-484.

5   Another Fat Soluble Vitamin

(a)   *Vitamin D*

If you live near the equator and spend an hour in the sun each day, you will have an adequate supply of vitamin D. Most of us don't. So take 800 units of vitamin D in the wintertime (either in your 1 tablespoon of cod liver oil, multivitamin or your calcium-vitamin D tablet). But in the summer, try to get some sun without burning please.

6   Effective Herbal Supplements

(a)   *Milk Thistle (Silymarin)*

Shown some effectiveness in chronic hepatitis including that is caused by alcohol[75] and Hepatitis C infection.[76] Effective dose is 140 mg of silymarin (the standardized extract) three times daily. No harmful effects have been reported.

(b)   *Saw palmetto and Stinging nettles*

Improvement in symptoms, urine flow volumes and residual urine volumes in patients with symptomatic enlargement of the prostate (BPH).[77] Effective dose of the 80-90% sterols extract (not just the dried berries) is 160mg twice daily. Do not continue taking the supplement if a positive effect is not seen within 3 months. May reduce PSA readings (the blood test for prostate cancer). Avoid taking for several weeks prior to having the PSA test done. The taking of Proscar (a drug with effects similar to saw palmetto) decreased the new cases of prostate cancer but appeared to increase death through more aggressive tumors. Therefore it is prudent to avoid both Proscar and saw palmetto unless the symptoms are severe enough to warrant the risk.

(c)   *Feverfew*

Reduces frequency of migraine headaches. Effective dose is 125 mg of the dried herb (2-3 leaves of fresh or dried leaves). This herb is easy to grow in a pot in the kitchen window or in the garden (it winters over).

---

[75] Canini F et al. Use of silymarin in the treatment of alcoholic hepatic steatosis. *Clin Ter* 1985;17:417-21.

[76] Liu JP; Manheimer E; Tsutani K; Gluud C Medicinal herbs for hepatitis C virus infection. *Cochrane Database Syst Rev* 2001;(4):CD003183.

[77] Bracher F. [Phytotherapy of benign prostatic hyperplasia] *Urologe* 1997,Jan 36(1):10-17.

(d)   *Black Cohosh*

Appears to function as an estrogen substitute. Effective dose is 20mg extract (Remifemin) 2 tablets twice daily.[78] May cause stomach upset. Do not take for longer than 6 months because unopposed estrogen is associated with cancer of the breast and uterus.

(e)   *Ginkgo*

Improves cognitive function in patients with Alzheimer's disease. Reduces muscle cramps. Reduces ringing in the ears.

(f)   *Capsicum*

Effective for chronic pain when applied topically. Thought to reduce Substance P in tissues which promotes pain. Use only on intact skin. Avoid use on inflamed tissues or open wounds (will burn the tissues).

(g)   *Melatonin*

Effective for jet lag when taken at bedtime for several days during and after travel. May reduce cataracts. Do not take if you have seasonal affective disorder (SAD). Patients with this disorder already have elevated melatonin levels.

(h)   *Garlic*

Crushed garlic is rich in allicin. Allicin has significant inhibitory effect against viruses, fungi and parasites. Known as Russian penicillin during World War 2 because of its widespread use for wound infections. May lower cholesterol although studies have been conflicting. May stimulate the immune system; monitor use in patients with autoimmune disorders. Inhibits blood clotting and therefore may reduce heart disease and stroke but also can promote bleeding. Avoid for one week prior to surgery.

(i)   *Valerian root*

Mild anti-anxiety effect; can be used for insomnia. Long-term regular use not recommended as tolerance and subsequent sleeplessness and anxiety can develop.

---

[78] Liske, E. Six-month randomized controlled trial of Remifemin. *Journal of Women's Health & Gender Based Medicine,* 11:2, 2002.

7   Herbal Supplements Not Recommended

(a)   *Echinacea*

Activates the immune system in an indiscriminate fashion. Although it may shorten the course of colds and flu, echinacea will exacerbate all autoimmune disorders including Multiple Sclerosis, Rheumatoid arthritis, pemphigus and others. Do not take for more than 8 weeks at a time for any reason.

(b)   *Glucosamine*

Has been shown to slow loss of cartilage in knee arthritis and some patients experienced some rebuilding of cartilage; it also reduces pain in knee arthritis. The problem is it can elevate blood sugars in patients with diabetes and patients taking glucosamine are more likely to develop diabetes (unmasking insulin resistance). Effective dose is 750-1000 mg twice daily (but follow your blood sugars).

(c)   *Kava-kava*

This is natural Xanax (which is the most habit-forming anti-anxiety drug) and has a significant withdrawal syndrome associated with excessive use. New Zealand has Kava clinics because of overuse of kava in the form of a concentrated tea.

8   Nutritional Supplements Considered Harmful and to be Avoided

(a)   *Iron*

Do not take iron if you are a man or a post-menopausal woman. Excess iron promotes disease of the liver, heart and pancreas. Excess iron may promote infections. Donate blood at the Red Cross when you have an opportunity (we were meant to have intestinal parasites to remove excess iron from our systems). Have your ferritin (blood iron level) checked by your doctor. Do not drink red wine if your iron level is elevated. You may take iron if you are pregnant or a menstruating woman with a low blood count. Most of us get adequate iron from our diets.

(b)   *Excessive doses of vitamin C*

Doses over 500 mg/day are associated with increased calcification of the blood vessels to the brain (which is associated with an increased risk of stroke). Vitamin C increases absorption of iron; do not take with a high iron meal (meat, fish or poultry).

(c) *Excessive doses of Beta-carotene*

Doses over 20,000 units per day are associated with an increased risk of lung cancer.

(d) *Excessive doses of zinc and copper*

Doses of more than 25 mg/day of zinc was associated with increased death in patients with AIDS (zinc deficiency is also associated with increased death). The recommended dose of zinc is 15mg per day, balanced by 2 mg of copper (the amount in most multivitamins). Excessive copper can also be harmful.

(e) *Excessive doses of DHEA-S*

The use of DHEA-S is associated with increased road-rage, as might be expected by the testosterone effect. I suggest trying the chromium and weight bearing exercise to 'rejuvenate' your hypothalamus and sex hormones.

(f) *Excessive doses of vitamin D*

Maximum recommended vitamin D is 800-1200 units/day although doses up to 2,000 units per day have not been found toxic. Most people unfortunately do not get adequate vitamin D from sun exposure. The cod liver oil has 800 units per tablespoon, which when added to our diet and lifestyle will ensure adequate vitamin D.

(g) *Borage oil*

May contain carcinogens and liver toxins

(h) *Ephedra*

Contains ephedrine, which is associated with cardiac deaths in patients using for weight loss.

(i) *Poke root*

Very toxic; causes low blood pressure, slow pulse and respiratory depression

(j) *Skullcap*

Can cause liver damage

9   One Daily without Iron

Choose a multi-vitamin that provides good levels of B vitamins without too much A or D. Most of the One Daily vitamins will have 400 units of vitamin D. Adequate vitamin D is important in the winter, as most of us do not have adequate sun exposure during the winter months.

Avoid iron-containing vitamins. Men and postmenopausal women do not need iron, and excess iron can be harmful.

The B vitamins lower homocysteine levels. Homocysteine damages blood vessels, oxidizes LDL cholesterol, and increases blood clotting which increases heart attacks and strokes. Lowering homocysteine levels reduces heart attacks, strokes, and blood clots. Most of us do not get adequate B vitamins, especially those over the age of 50 years old. Make sure your MVI has 25-50 mg of vitamin B-6, 25-50 mcg or more of vitamin B-12 and 400 mcg or more of folic acid (folate).

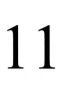

ULTIMATE SPORTS NUTRITION

(For the Ultimate Athlete hidden inside of you!)

1   The Cleaner and More Efficient Fuel

It is well known that trained athletes have a greater ability to burn fat,[79] which spares glycogen stores during endurance exercise. But is there a way to bypass training and get our bodies into great shape and endurance without spending all of that time exercising? Is there another way to get our bodies to burn fat as fuel from the get-go? Perhaps, so read on.

Using fat as fuel allows the heart muscle to be 25% more efficient while consuming 20% less oxygen. In fact, burning fat is like burning natural gas. The end products are carbon dioxide and water, which are easily excreted. Burning sugar requires more oxygen and produces more oxidative stress (read aging) as well as more toxic byproducts such as lactic acid, which leads to muscle fatigue and cellular stress (like using an unvented kerosene heater indoors?).

(a)   *Most of Our Energy is Stored as Fat*

Most of our energy is stored in fat: our body's energy stores (the average 70-kilogram man)
- Fat 12 kg   110,000 calories
- Protein 6 kg   24,000 calories
- Carbohydrate in muscle   0.4 kg   1,600 calories
- Carbohydrate in liver   0.07 kg   270 calories

While running a marathon the average runner will consume 1,000 calories per hour. It will take most people 3-4 hours to finish. This means that much of the energy used in running the marathon must come from stored fat. Hence the sensation of hitting the wall partway

---

[79] Pendergast DR, Leddy JJ, Venkatraman JT. *J Am Coll Nutr* 2000 Jun;19(3):345-50.

through as the runner must convert from glucose (glycogen or carbohydrate) to fat for fuel. But what if our bodies were primed to use fat as fuel from the beginning?

Mamo Wolde, the runner who won the 1968 Olympic marathon, was a hunter from sub-Saharan Africa who consumed mostly fat and protein from the animals he caught and ate. When asked about hitting the wall, he did not understand because he had never experienced such a feeling. He was able to run without developing fatigue. And at 36 years old he is the oldest person to ever win the Olympic marathon. So how do the rest of us develop this ability?

(b)   *You Need to Eat Fat to Burn Fat*

A high fat diet promotes increased fat utilization although it takes a period of adjustment for this to happen. Trained athletes have increased fat utilization during exercise even on a high carbohydrate diet (but I consider all of this training to be cheating- sort of). It appears to take more than one week on a high fat diet to change metabolism to increased fat metabolism during exercise. A positive effect is seen in athletes fed a high fat diet for 2-4 weeks (60-70% of calories from fat, 20-25% from protein, and the balance from carbohydrates). This must also be a very-low-carbohydrate diet.

Some studies (in mice, Greyhound dogs,[80] men and women[81]) have shown significant increases in speed and endurance. Many other studies have shown no difference. A few studies have shown a reduction in performance; most of these studies were of short duration (usually a week or less) which may reduce the body's ability to at least increase fat utilization during exercise. The general consensus is the high fat diet either improves or maintains aerobic capacity in cyclists, runners, Greyhound dogs, and mice.

No adverse affects on cardiovascular risk factors were seen in athletes on a high fat diet (70% of calories from fat). In fact, the good fats (HDL, LDL density and Apolipoprotein A) all went up, while the bad factors (LDL, triglycerides and Lipoprotein a) went down. All of this suggests an improvement of cardiovascular risk with the high fat diet.

2   Using Fat as Fuel Reduces Muscle Loss and Oxidative Stress

After an overnight fast much of our glycogen stores are depleted. The resting brain consumes 450-500 calories per day by itself. It normally uses glucose as the primary energy source. The glucose level in the blood is carefully maintained to support the brain. In early starvation, you deplete the glycogen stores in muscle and liver in order to maintain adequate blood glucose levels.

---

[80] Hill RC, Bloomberg MS et al. *Am J Vet Res* 2000 Dec:61(12):1566-73.
[81] Hoppeler H, Billeter R et al. *Int J Sports Med* 1999 Nov;20(8):522-6.

As fasting continues, your body begins to break down protein and fat to maintain the blood sugar. Initially you can lose up to one pound of muscle per day. But after a day or two, the ketoacids (the major one being beta-hydroxybutyrate) begin to accumulate from the breakdown of fat. Beta-hydroxybutyrate (one of the three ketoacids) inhibits the breakdown of muscle (blocks the proteases or enzymes that cause muscle breakdown).

(a) *You Gain Muscle While You Lose Only Fat*

The worst thing you can do to a fasting person is to give them a little bit of carbohydrate, which blocks all of the body's protective mechanisms (yet we do this in the hospitals with the glucose IV infusions). The same is true of people trying to lose weight: a little carbohydrate shuts down the production of beta-hydroxybutyrate and encourages the loss of protein from muscle to maintain blood sugar. The ketosis also reduces your appetite.

(b) *Reducing Calories Increases Health (and Happiness)*

Fasting lowers insulin and insulin-like growth factor-1 (IGF-1) and other markers of aging and tumor growth. Rodents fed a low calorie diet or alternate day feedings not only live longer, they are more resistant to developing brain-damaging diseases similar to Parkinson's and Alzheimer's diseases in response to brain toxins.

(c) *Beta-hydroxybutyrate: the Perfect Fuel for Reducing Aging and Maintaining Health*

Beta-hydroxybutyrate (the main fuel we produce as we burn fat on a very-low-carbohydrate diet) has many protective effects. It inhibits proteolysis (the breakdown of protein, thereby preventing the loss of muscle) and protects against oxygen deprivation (rats in ketosis survive 3-4 times longer than non-ketotic rats in a low oxygen environment). This reduced oxygen requirement could be very helpful in patients with stroke, heart attacks and other vascular injuries.

Beta-hydroxybutyrate is a more efficient source of energy than glucose; in the isolated rat heart preparation beta-hydroxybutyrate was shown to have the following effects: 25% increase in contractility and efficiency and a 20% decrease in oxygen consumption. It has also been shown to increase cellular energy production while simultaneously decreasing oxidative stress and cell damage. It is associated with increased levels of Coenzyme Q-10 production in the mitochondria and has been shown to reduce apoptosis (programmed cell death) and possibly aging.

3   What is a Ketogenic Diet?

A ketogenic diet is one in which your body uses fat as fuel instead of sugar. Seventy percent of your calories must be consumed as fat, with 15-25% as protein and 5-10% as carbohydrates. Within a few days your body begins to produce ketoacids including beta-hydroxybutyrate (BHB) which can efficiently fuel all cells in the body including the brain. You can check to see if you are burning fat (and therefore you are in ketosis) by checking your urine for ketones using Ketostix strips. All you need is trace to 1+ to effectively be burning fat.

(a)   *Why is burning fat instead of sugar good for your body?*

As discussed above, consuming less oxygen produces less oxidative stress. Burning fat as the major fuel improves cellular energy cycles with increased Coenzyme Q-10 levels and protection of mitochondrial DNA as well as less buildup of toxins in the body. Ketosis also protects the brain from the effects of low blood sugar (hypoglycemia) and low oxygen states (such as during stroke or heart attacks) which also may reduce aging.

The brain can use beta-hydroxybutyrate as the major fuel source during ketosis. This was shown in a study of subjects undergoing 30 days of starvation for weight loss (under medical supervision). During starvation, blood levels of beta-hydroxybutyrate were higher than glucose levels. When subjects were given an insulin infusion their blood sugars dropped to extremely low levels without central nervous system side effects. Beta-hydroxybutyrate levels were maintained despite the insulin infusion and protected against symptoms of hypoglycemia.

People who can be helped by the ketosis diet (the Mediterranean Hunter-Gatherer diet) include those with lung disease (reduced oxygen requirement), heart failure (improved cardiac efficiency), and multiple trauma victims (reduced oxidative stress and oxygen requirement). Other include patients needing weight loss, diabetes type 1 and 2 (reduced impact of hypoglycemia and improved weight loss) and children and adults with seizures. The ketosis diet is also being studied in patients with ADD, depression and bipolar disorders.

(b)   *What are the complications of the ketogenic diet?*

The ketogenic diet is not new. Pediatric neurologists have been using the ketogenic diet for 70 years without serious side effects in children with refractory seizures. Recent studies include patients with Rheumatoid arthritis, diabetes and heart disease as well as some psychiatric problems.

Constipation is one problem that can be seen, so drink more water and make sure you are getting enough fiber (20-30 grams per day is ideal). If you are not going to eat the green leafy vegetables such as kale, collards, mustard greens, cauliflower or broccoli, then you need to take a fiber supplement. Supplementing with magnesium also helps. The nuts have a fair amount of fiber but also have digestible carbohydrates.

Kidney stones are another problem so again drink more water (which prevents stone formation). There is no evidence that the ketogenic diet affects bone health in children or adults. There are no adverse affects on the kidneys and liver (this is not a high protein diet-only 15-25% calories are from protein).

(c) *What effect does the ketogenic diet have on risk factors for cardiovascular disease?*[82]

In most patients there is an improvement in cardiovascular risk factors as follows:
- Fasting serum insulin levels 34% lower (good)
- HDL increased 11% while LDL remained stable (good)
- LDL particle size became less dense (good)
- Lipoprotein (a) levels are lower (good)

In patients with diabetes and those with genetically high cholesterol (Familial Hyperlipidemia), the increased intake of cholesterol and saturated fat may raise cholesterol levels. In these patients it is important to monitor the LDL cholesterol levels after starting the ketogenic diet. As patients lose weight and as their diabetes improves or resolves, the LDL will drop back into a good range. In some patients I will start a lipid-lowering medication until we get the circumference of the waist down, with the plan of eventually stopping this medication as we meet our goals.

(d) *How do I eat a ketogenic diet?*

First, it is important to eat a well-balanced diet. Start the day with protein with healthy fat (no carbs)- Organic Italian Turkey Sausage or 3 eggs cooked "over easy" or "sunny side up" in olive oil or butter (or with organic turkey bacon). Take your supplements: chromium, magnesium, MSM, and cod liver oil (that's all you really need for the time being). The cod liver oil gives you healthy fat and helps balance the Omega 3/Omega 6 ratio of fats as well as all of the vitamin D you could need (don't take too much extra vitamin D, but the sun is ok).

Continue lunch with mostly protein with healthy fat (almost no carbs)- Tuna salad made with grape seed oil mayonnaise with celery. This will keep you in ketosis from morning

---

[82] Sharman MJ, Kraemer WJ et al. *Journal of Nutrition* 2002 Jul;132(7):1879-85.

to late afternoon. Add some nuts for a mid-afternoon snack- macadamia and Brazil nuts are the lowest in carbs.

For dinner have meat/fish/poultry with a salad/olive oil dressing and a low starch green leafy vegetable such as broccoli or mixed greens. Coffee is fine, but no sugar or half-and-half (a little heavy cream, however, is ok). A dry wine (1-2 glasses) or Miller Lite (1-2 cans) is acceptable (you'll have to not eat other carbs if you are going to stay in ketosis doing this).

Use Ketostix to see how you are doing (are you cheating too much or just enough?). These are urine dipsticks, which check your urine for ketones. You want to have a result of at least trace ketones. If you are negative for ketones, you pushed the envelope too hard with carbohydrates. Regroup and try it again.

(e)   *What foods do I eliminate?*

- Eliminate all grains (wheat, rice, oats, corn, barley, rye, etc) including all baked goods, breads and pasta, crackers. If it is made with flour, do not eat it.
- Eliminate all beans (mostly starch)
- Eliminate all potatoes, fries, chips, sweet potatoes, etc
- Eliminate most dairy (except heavy cream and butter)
- Eliminate all sugar
- Eliminate all sweet and dried fruit and fruit juices (one medium apple has more sugar than you can have in a whole day (equivalent to 8 glasses of wine!)
- Eliminate all processed foods (anything that comes in a package)

(f)   *How many grams of carbohydrate can I eat and still be in ketosis?*

Only you can determine what level will keep you in ketosis (that is why you check your urine for ketones as feedback). If you do not have ketones in your urine, you have eaten too many carbohydrates. A good rule is to try to stay less than 20 grams of digestible carbohydrate per day (not counting fiber).

If you want to gain a little weight, add more low sugar fruits. This is what the original hunter-gatherers did in the autumn, as all of the fruits became ripe in the fall. They would fatten up for the long winter of eating only meat and fat.

4   Isn't this Atkins' Diet?

(a)   *What is wrong with the Atkin's diet?*

The hormones and antibiotics in conventional meat and dairy products likely will cause other adverse health effects.

- Green leafy vegetables provide important nutrients. The diet can be designed to include these and still maintain ketosis.
- The consumption of nitrites in cured meats such as bacon and ham is highly associated with the development of colon cancer.
- The consumption of dairy products will worsen allergic symptoms and asthma in many people. Dairy should be avoided in all patients with asthma, recurrent sinusitis, frequent colds and bronchitis.
- Dr. Atkins provided the average person with an option for improving health in the real world of fast food. There are, however, better options to living well and feeling good.

(b)   *What is right about the Atkin's diet?*

The study at Duke using the Atkin's program has shown the following results:

- 95% of patients report more energy.
- 87% of patients report less heartburn.
- 85% of patients report improved mood.
- Average weight loss was 22 pounds.
- All parameters of heart disease risk improved: LDL-cholesterol levels dropped while HDL-cholesterol levels went up, triglycerides dropped and blood sugar levels improved.

Allergies are an Indication of Inflammation

Inflammation Leads to Heart Disease and Cancer

So Don't Ignore or Treat Your Allergies

Make Them Go Away

12

REASONS TO AVOID COW'S MILK

1   **Make Your Allergies and Asthma Go Away!**

(a)   *The Allergic Response*

In my clinical practice I have found food sensitivities to be much more common than I had ever expected. Milk, peanut, and wheat allergies are causing some of the allergic rhinitis, asthma, and rashes that I see. Patients have been able to stop 2 or even 3 prescription drugs after eliminating offending items, then developing symptoms again when re-challenging themselves.

(b)   *Much of our allergies and asthma are related directly to the food we eat*

When our son was five years old, he developed asthma (both my wife and I had asthma as children). We cleaned the house, took out the rugs, and put in the HEPA filters. He got better and then worse again. He was diagnosed with pneumonia twice and had chronic congestion and a nocturnal cough. He was using two inhalers. Nothing we did seemed to make much difference.

One of my patients had suggested I buy the book Optimal Wellness by Ralph Golan, M.D. He said it had good sections on hypoglycemia and food allergies. Twice I went to buy the book and twice I left without it because the information seemed so foreign. I was reluctant because if Dr. Golan was right, then I was ignorant of (and resistant to) what he was suggesting.

I finally did buy the book. Dr. Golan suggests that at least some of asthma and allergies are on the basis of food allergies. Our son John (who was now six years old) and I went to an organic food store and bought the foods that Dr. Golan suggested we substitute for our usual diet (John and I did this together). Over the next two weeks John's cough, congestion, and wheezing went away. As we added foods back, John began coughing after eating peanut butter crackers. When we got to milk, his eyes began burning and he cried. John is now eleven years old and has put his inhalers away ever since changing his diet. And this was a kid who had lived on all the foods he was allergic to, including string cheese, yogurt, cereal with milk, ice cream, pizza, macaroni and cheese, and peanut butter crackers.

Most people will notice that drinking milk gives them more mucus. Singers are told to avoid milk before concerts to reduce congestion. Athletes are told to avoid all milk products before sporting events to reduce secretions. What are our bodies telling us by this? Don't drink milk.

(c)   *How do foods cause allergic symptoms?*

It appears that large proteins absorbed through our gut stimulate our immune system and initiate much of the allergic response we see in the upper and lower respiratory tracts. The large proteins in milk and peanuts had apparently stimulated our son's immune system to react to dust, mold, and animal dander in his local environment. We could not eliminate the dust, mold, mildew, and mouse dander adequately from our old house but we could modify his diet, which in his case has done the trick.

And this trick has worked over and over again in my patients. The most common offenders are milk proteins (casein and lactalbumin), wheat protein (gluten), and peanuts, as well as the sulfites in wine, and the proteins in orange juice and corn. My patients report that they have stopped all of their allergy and/or asthma medications and only need them if they cheat (i.e. Pizza and ice cream in milk-allergic, or flour-based products in wheat-allergic).

One patient with this was a surgeon from Europe in his mid thirties with a history of asthma since childhood. He was very doubtful, but after he eliminated the twelve most common foods that cause an allergic response, his asthma was gone. When he again tried wheat, orange juice and red wine (using the elimination and reintroduction diet), his asthma symptoms returned. Since avoiding these, his asthma has resolved and he no longer needs his inhalers (and his peak flow is normal).

The former chairman of Pediatrics at The Johns Hopkins School of Medicine authored a book entitled <u>Don't Drink Your Milk</u> (by Dr. Oski). He reported on his significant clinical experience that milk, wheat, peanut, oranges, wine, etc. initiate an abnormal immune response in many individuals causing recurrent ear infections, asthma, and gastrointestinal problems. More on the elimination diet later.

(d)   *Don't Drink Your Milk (if you have allergies, asthma, or head congestion)*

The Dairy Council has done a wonderful job of marketing milk as an important calcium source. The Harvard Nurses Health study showed that the more milk women drank, the more fractures they had (in this study of 74,000 women, the women who drank three glasses of milk per day had more fractures than those who rarely drank milk did). There are many healthier calcium sources, such as the green leafy vegetables and sardines, etc. If you aren't going to base your major calorie intake on green leafy vegetables, then I suggest one or two calcium/ magnesium supplements per day (see chapter on Nutritional Supplements).

Milk has also been associated with ovarian cancer, juvenile-onset diabetes mellitus, and cataracts. I encourage my patients with allergies and those feeling less than great to eliminate milk. Eliminating wheat (wheat flour-based foods) is also healthier for many people. This consists of eating a whole food diet, eliminating all processed and packaged foods that you cannot identify the contents.

2   **The Most Common Foods Associated with Symptoms of Sensitivity**

- Headaches: wheat, chocolate, MSG, nuts, wine, cheese, eggs, milk, citrus fruits
- Allergic rhinitis (hayfever): milk, wheat, peanuts, chocolate, sulfites in wine
- Hives: strawberries, tomatoes, chocolate, eggs, shellfish, mangoes, pork, peanuts, nuts
- Asthma: milk, wheat, tartrazine (FDA yellow dye #5), aspirin, peanuts, orange juice, sulfites in wine, wine vinegar and Balsamic vinegar
- Hyperactivity, poor attention: corn, wheat, milk, soybeans, beer (grains- hops, barley)
- Eczema: eggs, citrus fruits, tomatoes

(a)   *Milk Makes More Mucus (so does wine, orange juice, and chocolate)*

Milk allergy and asthma is a well-known association in children. Athletes and singers are consistently told to avoid milk products before important engagements because they often increase airway congestion and secretions. So why do we encourage people to consume a substance otherwise foreign to their existence after weaning (for the USDA and the economy of course!)? Contrary to the popular belief that we outgrow our allergy to milk as we grow older, it can manifest itself in different ways in adults. These can include allergic rhinitis, chronic fatigue and chronic low-grade depression. I have seen many patients (including my six year old son and a 35 year old surgeon from Denmark) have their symptoms resolve completely following the exclusion of the offending food, most commonly milk, wheat, sulfites and peanuts.

(b) *Milk Products Are Everywhere* *(and take an effort to avoid)*

- Milk, cheese, yogurt, ice cream
- Cream in your coffee (the hardest for me to give up), Lattes
- Pizza
- Bagel and cream cheese
- Cottage cheese
- Baked goods with casein (the milk protein that promotes allergy)
- Protein drinks with casein
- Any food with casein listed on the ingredients
- Lactaid products still have the allergenic proteins

(c) *What are the options?*

- Fresh or frozen berries in a smoothie (with heavy cream?) for dessert instead of ice cream
- What?! For pizza? Is there no acceptable substitute? Won't the anchovies protect me?

3   The Allergy-Addiction Connection

The allergic response to foods causes the release of adrenaline and endorphins (morphine-like substances) that give us an energy boost and a greater sense of well being and creativity. This can be followed by a crash. If the suspected allergen is not eaten we can get a mild withdrawal reaction making us crave the food. The foods we crave (even if the craving is very subtle) can be the very foods making us feel less than great to begin with (causing fatigue and depressed mood). Common substances associated with this reaction are listed below. You may not want to release your substance, but at least you will understand your body and it's reaction.

Foods associated with Allergy-Addiction.

Alcoholic beverages, particularly beer and wine
Chocolate, Coffee, Tobacco
Corn, wheat, and other grains

People can tend to binge on these substances because of the heightened sense of well being and productivity, making elimination difficult. If these substances are also causing significant head congestion, asthma, headaches, or eczema, it may be worth the decreased productivity for a more livable life.

218

4   The Other Side of Soy

Patients told me not to recommend soy. Soy contains substances that can promote abnormal thyroid growth and goiter. There are substances that interfere with protein digestion. In addition, the acid-extraction procedure that is used to process soymilk and tofu oxidizes and hydrolyzes the proteins. Fermented soy products (Miso), in contrast, are ok because these are not acid-extracted and the bacteria break down the substances that cause the above problems. Consider almond-milk or rice-milk although these are very high in carbs.

5   The Food Rotation Diet

Eating the same foods habitually may also stimulate the immune system. It is good to vary your diet. Small amounts of irritating foods eaten intermittently are much less likely to cause a problem. But if you already have developed sensitivity, complete avoidance for several weeks to months may be required to reduce the reaction and allow health to return.

Allergy Elimination Diet

You may eat the following:
- Most fruits, except citrus
- Most vegetables, except corn, tomatoes, potatoes, eggplant
- Brown or white rice
- Turkey
- White fish-flounder, sole, halibut
- Almonds, walnuts, sunflower seeds

Avoid the following:
- All wheat products
- All dairy products

All foods you think you might be sensitive to: especially peanuts, certain nuts, eggs, chocolate, banana, mango, pork, beef, chicken, beer, wine, yeast, or potatoes.

Of 367 asthmatic children, 257 had a history of symptoms triggered by specific foods. Double blind, placebo controlled oral food challenges confirmed 63% of them. Wheat, eggs, soy, nuts, dairy were the most common triggers.[83]

---

[83] Bock SA. In: Tinkelman DG, Naspitz CK, eds. *Childhood Asthma: Pathophysiology and Treatment.* New York: Marcel Dekker; 1993:537-551.

If You Are Living in the Desert,

Eat Grains

Otherwise, Avoid the Pasta and Bread

13

WHAT'S WRONG WITH WHEAT

1   There is no Wheat or Corn in the Mediterranean Hunter-Gatherer Diet

Why would I suggest we eliminate wheat from our diet? Could it be because pasta and bread are quickly metabolized to simple sugars and rapidly raise blood sugar and insulin levels? Or is that some of my patients get headaches and asthma from wheat? Or that not eating wheat is associated with lower blood pressure in some patients. Some people are as attached to their pasta and bread as the alcoholic is to his alcohol? Sure, but I find the following studies to be both interesting and disturbing:

(a)   *Wheat gluten (the protein in wheat) promotes the development of diabetes in mice*

Mice bred to develop non-obese diabetes (NOD mice) who were fed a gluten free diet developed diabetes much less frequently (only 15% did, compared to 64% on a diet containing gluten). And the 15% who did develop diabetes did so at a much older age (244 days vs. 197 days- a long time for a mouse). Both groups were fed the same milk protein and vitamin content.[84]

In mice and pigs (*we are genetically very similar to pigs*), gluten binds to the insulin receptors; at low levels gluten increases glucose utilization (weight gain), at higher levels gluten inhibits glucose utilization (insulin resistance).

(b)   *So why am I worried about some mice and pigs?*

Seven to ten percent of patients with type 1 diabetes (the type similar to NOD mice) have celiac disease (gluten sensitive enteropathy- inflammation of the intestine due to

---

[84] Funda DP, Kaas A, Bock T, Tlaskalova-Hogenova H, Buschard K. Gluten-free diet prevents diabetes in NOD mice. *Diabetes Metab Res Rev* 1999 Sep-Oct;15(5):323-7.

sensitivity to wheat protein). Only 1/100-200 people without type 1 diabetes have celiac disease.[85] Eleven percent of patients with untreated Celiac disease have autoantibodies against the pancreatic islet cells (the cells that produce insulin; their destruction produces diabetes). These autoantibodies often disappear with the avoidance of gluten. (fourteen percent have autoantibodies against the thyroid, many of whom develop thyroid disease).[91]

Fifty-three percent of untreated patients with Celiac disease have autoantibodies, while only 20% of treated patients (avoiding wheat gluten) have autoantibodies (i.e. autoimmunity improves or resolves off wheat). What is interesting is that it appears we may be able to calm the immune system by changing our diet.

The reason this is important is because NOD mice treated with anti T-cell therapy (eliminates the immune cells that destroy pancreatic cells) regrow their pancreatic islet cells and no longer have diabetes (amazing- the potential to regrow islet cells is not lost!!! The immune system is just suppressing their growth).

Summary: If you have diabetes, thyroid disease, or other autoimmune disorder, it is probably a good idea to avoid wheat gluten.

(c) *Wheat and Crohn's disease (another inflammatory bowel disease)*

Cereals (wheat and corn) and dairy products have been shown to worsen Crohn's disease, and the elimination of these improves all parameters. In refractory patients that are unresponsive even to high dose steroids, an elemental diet produces remission in 90% of these patients.[86]

Dietary lectins (proteins of grains-particularly corn and wheat) have been associated with bowel inflammation and the promotion of autoimmune diseases including Rheumatoid arthritis. It has been shown that removal of the bowel inflammation improves the other manifestations of autoimmunity.[87]

(d) *Gluten Exorphin A-5 is a morphine-like substance from wheat gluten*

Could the eating of wheat actually be addictive? No wonder patients complain if you try to take away their pasta and bread.

---

[85] Ventura A, Neri E, Ughi C, Leopaldi A, Citta A, Not T.J Gluten-dependent diabetes-related and thyroid-related autoantibodies in patients with celiac disease. *Pediatr* 2000 Aug;137(2):263-5.

[86] Hunter JO. Nutritional factors in inflammatory bowel disease. *Eur J Gastroenterol Hepatol* 1998 Mar;10(3):235-7.
[87] Cordain L, Toohey L, Smith MJ, Hickey MS. Modulation of immune function by dietary lectins in rheumatoid arthritis. *Br J Nutr* 2000 Mar;83(3):207-17.

Gluten Exorphin A-5 is an opioid (morphine-like) peptide sequence of 5 amino acids, which recurs 15 times in each molecule of gluten. It is released by protein digestion in the stomach and small intestine. Both oral and intravenous A-5 produce central and peripheral nervous system effects on learning and response similar to narcotics. These effects also seen in gluten feed mice (i.e. digestion release these exorphins which are then absorbed). Effects blocked by narcotic antagonists (medications that block the effects of narcotics).

There is an association of gluten intolerance and autoantibodies with schizophrenia, psychosis, and degeneration of the part of our brain which controls balance (the cerebellum).[88]

(e)   *Wheat and Colon Cancer*

The consumption of certain food groups is associated with increased colorectal cancer in Italy and France (countries that pride themselves on their pasta and bread).[89] [90] Look below at Table 13-1. The people who ate the most cereal, rice and bread had a doubling of their risk of colorectal cancer. A risk of 2.0 suggests a doubling of risk. A risk of 1.7 suggests a 70% increase in risk.

---

[88] Harper DN, Nisbet RH, Siegert RJ. Dietary gluten and learning to attend to redundant stimuli in rats. *Biol Psychiatry* 1997 Dec 1;42(11):1060-6.
[89] Franceschi S, Favero A, La Vecchia C, Negri E, Conti E, Montella M, Giacosa A, Nanni O, Decarli A. Food groups and risk of colorectal cancer in Italy. *Int J Cancer* 1997 Jul 3;72(1):56-61.
[90] Boutron-Ruault MC, Senesse P, Faivre J, Chatelain N, Belghiti C, Meance S. Foods as risk factors for colorectal cancer: a case-control study in Burgundy (France). *Eur J Cancer Prev* 1999 Jul;8(3):229-35.

TABLE 13-1

The Association of Wheat and Other Foods with Colorectal Cancer

Italy (risk ratio)	France (risk ratio)	Food Group (from highest to lowest risk foods)
	2.4	Deli meats (People who ate the most deli meats had 140% more colon cancer than the average person in France)
1.7	2.0	Cereals, rice, bread (Large consumers of starches had 70-100% more cancer than average in Italy and France)
1.4		Refined sugar (Excess sugar consumers had 40% more cancer)
1.2		Potatoes (Excess potatoes increased risk by 20%)
1.1		Cakes and desserts (Great consumers of cakes had 10% more cancer)
1.0	1.0	Fresh meat (Excess intake of meat did not change cancer risk)
1.0		Alcohol (Alcohol intake did not seem to help or hurt on average)
0.7	1.0	Fish (A suggestion of possible decrease in cancer risk if you eat a lot of fish)
0.7		Fresh fruit other than citrus (Consuming more fruit was much safer than consuming more sugar and starches)
0.6	0.3	Raw or cooked vegetables (The people who ate the most of their vegetables had 40-70% less cancer than average- sign me up!)

The people who ate the most raw or cooked vegetables had a 30% to 70% reduction in colorectal cancer. A risk of less than 1.0 suggests a reduction in risk of colon cancer (fish, fruits, vegetables). There were 20% fewer colon cancers in people who ate one serving of vegetables per day.

There was only a slight increased risk in patients who ate the most cakes and desserts. So it appears you can have your cake and eat it too, but just not the pasta and bread (I would stick to oatmeal-raisin cookies).

(f) *Other cancers are also promoted by a high starch and sugar diet*

The Harvard Nurses Health Study has confirmed these findings in that pancreatic cancer occurred four times as often in the women who ate the most rice and potatoes. Pancreatic cancer, breast cancer, prostate cancer and colon cancer have all been shown to be promoted by a high sugar/starch diet.

Could the consumption of wheat flour promote?

- Diabetes
- Inflammatory bowel disease
- Celiac disease
- Irritable bowel syndrome
- Colorectal cancer
- Schizophrenia

Studies referenced below suggest this may be true.

Cordain L, Miller JB, Eaton SB, Mann N, Holt SH, Speth JD. Plant-animal subsistence ratios and macronutrient energy estimations in worldwide hunter-gatherer diets. *Am J Clin Nutr* 2000 Mar;71(3):682-92.

Both anthropologists and nutritionists have long recognized that the diets of modern-day hunter-gatherers may represent a reference standard for modern human nutrition and a model for defense against certain diseases of affluence. Because the hunter-gatherer way of life is now probably extinct in its purely un-Westernized form, nutritionists and anthropologists must rely on indirect procedures to reconstruct the traditional diet of preagricultural humans. In this analysis, we incorporate the most recent ethnographic compilation of plant-to-animal economic subsistence patterns of hunter-gatherers to estimate likely dietary macronutrient intakes (% of energy) for environmentally diverse hunter-gatherer populations. Furthermore, we show how differences in the percentage of body fat in prey animals would alter protein intakes in hunter-gatherers and how a maximal protein ceiling influences the selection of other macronutrients.

Our analysis showed that whenever and wherever it was ecologically possible, hunter-gatherers consumed high amounts (45-65% of energy) of animal food. Most (73%) of the worldwide hunter-gatherer societies derived >50% (> or =56-65% of energy) of their subsistence from animal foods, whereas only 14% of these societies derived >50% (> or =56-65% of energy) of their subsistence from gathered plant foods. This high reliance on animal-based foods coupled with the relatively low carbohydrate content of wild plant foods produces universally characteristic macronutrient consumption ratios in which protein is elevated (19-35% of energy) at the expense of carbohydrates (22-40% of energy).

Funda DP, Kaas A, Bock T, Tlaskalova-Hogenova H, Buschard K. Gluten-free diet prevents diabetes in NOD mice. *Diabetes Metab Res Rev* 1999 Sep-Oct;15(5):323-7.

Epidemiological as well as animal studies have shown that environmental factors such as nutrition contribute to the development of diabetes. In this study we investigated whether the early introduction of a gluten-free diet can influence the onset and/or incidence of diabetes, as well as insulitis and the number of gut mucosal lymphocytes, in non-obese diabetic (NOD) mice. METHODS: Gluten-free and standard Altromin diets (with the same milk protein and vitamin content) were given to breeding pairs of NOD mice as well as to the first generation of NOD female mice, which were then observed for 320 days.

RESULTS: A substantially lower diabetes incidence (chi(2)=15.8, p=0.00007) was observed in NOD mice on the gluten-free diet (15%, n=27) compared to mice on the standard diet (64%, n=28). In addition, mice on the gluten-free diet developed diabetes significantly later (244+/-24 days SEM) compared to those on the standard diet (197+/-8 days, p=0.03). No differences in the number of CD3(+), TCR-gammadelta(+), IgA(+), and IgM(+) cells in the small intestine were observed.

CONCLUSION: We showed that gluten-free diet both delayed and to a large extent prevented diabetes in NOD mice that have never been exposed to gluten.

Ventura A, Neri E, Ughi C, Leopaldi A, Citta A, Not T. Gluten-dependent diabetes-related and thyroid-related autoantibodies in patients with celiac disease. *Pediatr* 2000 Aug;137(2):263-5.

Patients with celiac disease are at high risk of having autoimmune disorders. Moreover, untreated patients with celiac disease have been found to have a higher than expected prevalence of organ-specific autoantibodies. In a prospective study of 90 patients with celiac disease, we found that the prevalence of diabetes and thyroid-related serum antibodies was 11.1% and 14.4%, respectively. Like antiendomysium autoantibodies, these organ-specific antibodies seem to be gluten-dependent and tend to disappear during a gluten-free diet.

De Vitis I, Ghirlanda G, Gasbarrini G. Prevalence of coeliac disease in type I diabetes: a multicentre study. *Acta Paediatr Suppl* 1996 May;412:56-7.

The aim of this study was to point out the prevalence ratio and the clinical presentation of coeliac disease (CD) in a large group of insulin-dependent diabetes mellitus (IDDM) patients. PATIENTS AND METHODS: 1114 patients affected by IDDM were screened for CD using antigliadin and antiendomysium antibodies. Patients who were positive for at least one test underwent an endoscopic biopsy of the descending duodenum in order to verify the presence of villous atrophy. Subjects with CD started a gluten-free diet and underwent a clinical follow up.

RESULTS: Villous atrophy was found in 63 patients (5.6%). Among the Italian population, the rate was 7%. Twenty-four percent of coeliac patients presented with diarrhea, while 22% were completely symptom-free. A significant correlation was found between the presence of villous atrophy and the duration and onset of diabetes.

CONCLUSIONS: The prevalence of CD in IDDM is higher than previously reported, although the ratio range in different centers from 1.7 to 10%, probably due to both environmental and genetic factors. Twenty-two percent of coeliac patients were completely symptom-free. The prevalence seems to be significantly related to the duration and onset of IDDM.

Cordain L, Toohey L, Smith MJ, Hickey MS. Modulation of immune function by dietary lectins in rheumatoid arthritis. *Br J Nutr* 2000 Mar;83(3):207-17.

Despite the almost universal clinical observation that inflammation of the gut is frequently associated with inflammation of the joints and vice versa, the nature of this relationship remains elusive. In the present review, we provide evidence for how the interaction of dietary lectins with enterocytes and lymphocytes may facilitate the translocation of both dietary and gut-derived pathogenic antigens to peripheral tissues, which in turn causes persistent peripheral antigenic stimulation. In genetically susceptible individuals, this antigenic stimulation may ultimately result in the expression of overt rheumatoid arthritis (RA) via molecular mimicry, a process whereby foreign peptides, similar in structure to endogenous peptides, may cause antibodies or T-lymphocytes to cross-react with both foreign and endogenous peptides and thereby break immunological tolerance.

By eliminating dietary elements, particularly lectins, which adversely influence both enterocyte and lymphocyte structure and function, it is proposed that the peripheral antigenic stimulus (both pathogenic and dietary) will be reduced and thereby result in a diminution of disease symptoms in certain patients with RA.

Franceschi S, Favero A, La Vecchia C, Negri E, Conti E, Montella M, Giacosa A, Nanni O, Decarli A. Food groups and risk of colorectal cancer in Italy. *Int J Cancer* 1997 Jul 3;72(1):56-61.

The proportion of colorectal cancer attributed to dietary habits is high, but several inconsistencies remain, especially with respect to the influence of some food groups. To further elucidate the role of dietary habits, 1,225 subjects with cancer of the colon, 728 with cancer of the rectum and 4,154 controls, hospitalized with acute non-neoplastic diseases, were interviewed between 1992 and 1996 in 6 different Italian areas. The validated food-frequency questionnaire included 79 questions on food items and recipes, categorized into 16 food groups.

After allowance for non-dietary confounding factors and total energy intake, significant trends of increasing risk of colorectal cancer with increasing intake emerged for bread and cereal dishes (odds ratio [OR] in highest vs. lowest quintile = 1.7), potatoes (OR = 1.2), cakes and desserts (OR = 1.1), and refined sugar (OR = 1.4). Intakes of fish (OR = 0.7), raw and cooked vegetables (OR = 0.6 for both) and fruit other than citrus fruit (OR = 0.7) showed a negative association with risk. Consumption of eggs and meat (white, red or processed meats) seemed uninfluential. Most findings were similar for colon and rectum, but some negative associations (i.e., coffee and tea, and fish) appeared stronger for colon cancer.

Our findings lead us to reconsider the role of starchy foods and refined sugar in light of recent knowledge on the digestive physiology of carbohydrates and the insulin/colon cancer hypothesis. The beneficial role of most vegetables is confirmed, with more than 20% reduction in risk of colorectal cancer from the addition of one daily serving.

Boutron-Ruault MC, Senesse P, Faivre J, Chatelain N, Belghiti C, Meance S. Foods as risk factors for colorectal cancer: a case-control study in Burgundy (France*). Eur J Cancer Prev* 1999 Jul;8(3):229-35.

Although the high meat-low vegetable diet is considered the reference high-risk diet for colorectal cancer, particularly in USA communities, other at-risk dietary patterns, such as high intakes of processed meat and refined carbohydrates are emerging. Little is known about risk factors for colorectal cancer in France, a country at high risk of rectal cancer and moderately high risk of colon cancer. We compared diet of colorectal cancer cases (n = 171) and general population controls (n = 309) in Burgundy (France). Categories of intake were established by sex and based on the distributions of food intakes in controls.

Odds ratios for the fourth Vs first quartile of intake (OR4) were 2.0 (1.1-3.6) for refined cereal products (rice, pasta and pastry), 2.4 (1.3-4.5) for delicatessen, 2.3 (1.2-4.2) for pates, 1.7 (1.1-2.8) for offal and 2.1 (1.1-4.0) for butter, lard and cream. There was no association with consumption of fresh meat (OR4 = 1.2), fish (OR4 = 1.5), egg (OR4 = 1.1) or dairy products (OR4 = 1.0). A protective effect of vegetables was only observed for left colon cancer (OR3 = 0.3; 0.1-0.6). In men, the most significant risk factors were refined cereal products, seasoning animal fats, chocolate and coffee, whereas risk factors were delicatessen, fat meat, pasta, rice, and chocolate in women.

The strong association with refined cereal products is consistent with the hypothesis of a role of hyperinsulinism in colorectal carcinogenesis. The association with processed but not fresh meat suggests the importance of exogenous carcinogenesis in that area.

Deneo-Pellegrini H, De Stefani E, Ronco A. Vegetables, fruits, and risk of colorectal cancer: a case-control study from Uruguay. *Nutr Cancer* 1996;25(3):297-304.

To examine whether vegetable and fruit intake modify colorectal cancer risk, a case-control study was conducted in Uruguay. Dietary patterns were assessed in detail (for cases before diagnosis or symptoms occurred) by use of a food frequency questionnaire on 61 food items, which allowed the calculation of total energy intake. Nutrient residuals were calculated through regression analysis. After adjustment for potential confounders (which included body mass index, total energy, and total alcohol intake), a reduction in risk for total vegetable intake, total fruit intake, and lettuce, apple, and banana consumption was observed. The strongest protection was observed for banana intake (odds ratio 0.28; 95% confidence level 0.16-0.50) for consumption in the third tertile compared with the first.

Hunter JO. Nutritional factors in inflammatory bowel disease.

Eur J Gastroenterol Hepatol 1998 Mar;10(3):235-7.

During the past 20 years there has been growing interest in the importance of nutritional factors in the pathogenesis of inflammatory bowel disease. There are so far no definite links between ulcerative colitis and diet, but both epidemiologists and clinicians have studied links with Crohn's disease. Epidemiological studies, although retrospective, have suggested that patients with Crohn's disease eat more sugar and sweets that control individuals; however, when dietary sugar is restricted, there is little clinical benefit. The clinical approach to nutrition in Crohn's disease has been by the use of elemental diets, which will produce symptomatic and objective remission in up to 90% of compliant patients. Those who return to normal eating soon relapse but, in some studies, have enjoyed prolonged remission on exclusion diets.

The foods excluded have been not sugar, **but predominantly cereals, dairy products and yeast**. Attention has now switched to the possible harmful role of fat in Crohn's disease. The efficacy of elemental feeds appears to depend not on the presentation of nitrogen but on the amount of long chain triglyceride present. Increases in recent years in the frequency of Crohn's disease in Japan have been correlated with increased dietary fat intake, and a recent study suggested that W-3 fatty acids, which are metabolized by immunomodulatory leukotrienes and prostaglandins, may have a beneficial role to play. The links between nutrition and Crohn's disease have now become strong and the role of fat may be the most exciting of all.

A Little Alcohol Appears to be Good

More is not Better

A Lot is Definitely Bad

14

THE MODERATE DRINKING OF ALCOHOL

1 Paths of Escape

When in the course of life we find ourselves feeling trapped by our circumstances and choices, is it not ok to try to take the pressure off by opening up potential options for a temporary escape?

- To allow us to keep our commitments.
- To allow us to stay interdependent without losing our minds.

(a) *What are the potential paths of escape?*

- Exercise, be it jogging, walking the dog, tennis, yoga, Tai Chi, etc. are excellent and natural ways of releasing endorphins and increasing our sense of well-being and fitness.
- Reading to escape to new and different worlds (*But who will empty the dishwasher?*).
- Working all the time is effective but may remove us too much from our interdependence.
- Cigarettes can take the edge off (*by releasing endorphins and adrenaline*) but are destructive to our tissues and promote aging.
- Cheating on your spouse is also destructive and to be avoided (*But can we flirt just a little, please?*).
- Narcotics and cocaine are much too potent (*Animals will choose cocaine over food until they starve to death*). Avoid at all costs.
- A little apple cider.

(b) *A Little Apple Cider*

Johnny Appleseed (*John Chapman was his real name*) introduced apple trees to much of the new world along the Ohio River in the early 19th century. But the trees he propagated produced small tart apples suitable only for making cider, which then fermented to hard cider (*alcohol content of 5% or a little more*). And each homestead was required by land grant to set out at least fifty apple or pear trees. This meant that each farm was capable of producing 2,000 gallons of cider per year (*for personal use?*). Due to the pollution of the rivers, often the cider was the safest thing to drink, even for the young people. The puritans approved of cider because it came from the American apple rather than the sinful grape.

It was not until this century that we began planting grafted apple trees capable of producing the sweet apples we know today. In fact, all Granny Smith apples have come from the same tree, which has been reproduced by taking a small twig and grafting it onto a stem of another apple tree. The few apple varieties we have now were selected for their high sugar contents. Granny Smith apples are now the closest apple you can get to the original American apples (*in terms of tartness*) except for crabapples and wild apples. But don't eat too many modern apples because they are loaded with sugar (*by design*).

(c)   *The Good of Alcohol*

But getting back to alcohol, there is much evidence associating the moderate use of alcohol (*see definition below*) with increased longevity and decreased heart disease. Alcohol intake is associated with a decreased incidence of coronary heart disease (*heart attacks*) among men and women and among patients with diabetes and those with previous heart attacks or heart failure. Moderate alcohol consumption appears to inhibit IL-6 production or activity (*Interleukin-6 induces an inflammatory response promoting blood clotting and vessel wall damage leading to heart disease and strokes*). This could partly explain the protective effect.

Regular alcohol consumption has an insulin-sensitizing effect on skeletal muscle that down-regulates insulin secretion. Since excess insulin promotes heart disease, this may further explain the protective effect. Women, who drink alcohol regularly and moderately, tend to have a decidedly lower body-mass index (*BMI*) than non-drinking women, despite slightly higher caloric intakes do. And we know that lower waist circumference is associated with a lower risk of breast cancer.

The consumption of red wine is associated with decreased cancer. But could this be explained by the demographic fact that people in this country who drink wine are richer and therefore receive better disease prevention and early detection? The cardiac protective effect is seen with all types of alcohol and all demographic groups.

Alcohol reduces the liver's production of sugar and thereby lowers blood sugars in patients with diabetes (and the rest of us as well). This is a good thing unless you are taking insulin or medications which increase insulin levels (*glipizide, glyburide, etc; see the diabetes chapter for details*).

What is this? A doctor who advocates drinking alcohol?! Do not drink if you have or have had a problem with alcohol or other drugs.

(d) *Do not drink if you have or have had the problem with alcohol or other drugs*

Yes, alcohol is a drug. Drinking alcohol lowers your blood sugar and insulin levels by reducing gluconeogenesis (the liver production of sugar). Alcohol increases metabolic rate and thereby women who drink alcohol consume more calories but weigh less than women who do not drink. Consumption of moderate amounts of alcohol is associated with improved blood sugars in patients with diabetes. Is also associated with much less cardiac death in patients with diabetes and also less congestive heart failure (unless abused).

Yes, alcohol is a drug. It impairs judgement, lowers inhibitions, impairs your ability to drive an automobile and can damage your liver, heart, pancreas and brain with chronic excessive use. Drinking alcohol can lead to dependence and considerable social disruption including loss of your job, your marriage, your driver's license and may lead to death for you and others.

Alcohol is a two-edged sword. Ok, let's say you have diabetes or Syndrome X and you want the benefits of alcohol without the risks (or you just do not want to drink). What are your options? Another drug very similar to alcohol is metformin (Glucophage-Greek for consumes sugar). It is associated with a reduction in cardiac death, reduces the liver production of sugar, helps people lose weight and has been shown to delay the onset of diabetes when used in obese adolescents.

2 Moderation Management

But the protective effects are only seen with moderate drinking and disappear with excessive drinking. There is a group called Moderation Management that has put together some guidelines to help us make healthy decisions about drinking alcohol.

(a) *Definition of Moderate Drinking:*

- Men: Up to 3-4/day for 3 or 4 days of the week with a maximum of fourteen drinks per week
- Women: Up to 2-3/day for 3 or 4 days of the week with a maximum of nine drinks per week
- By the way, these are limits and not targets.

(b) *A Moderate Drinker:*

- Considers an occasional drink to be a small, though enjoyable, part of life
- Has hobbies, interests, and other ways to relax and enjoy life that do not involve alcohol
- Usually has friends who are moderate drinkers or nondrinkers
- Generally has something to eat before, during, or soon after drinking
- Usually does not drink for longer than an hour or two on any particular occasion
- Usually does not drink faster than one drink per half-hour
- Usually does not exceed the 0.055% blood alcohol content drinking limit
- Feels comfortable with his or her use of alcohol (*never drinks secretly and does not spend a lot of time thinking about drinking or planning to drink*)
- Never drives under the influence of alcohol

(c) *Definition of a drink:*

- 5 oz. of wine (*no topping up please*)
- 1.5 oz. of whiskey/liquor
- 12 oz. regular beer
- 18 oz. of light beer.

But watch the carbohydrates in beer. Regular beer has 13-18 grams of carbohydrate; Sam Adams Light has 10 grams; Coors Light and Amstel Light each have 5 grams; Miller Lite has 3.2 grams; Michelob Ultra has 2.2 grams

(d) *Alcoholics are often very spiritual people; they just have the wrong spirit.*

The Moderation Management group also recommends abstaining from drinking for 30 days to define your relationship with alcohol. If you have difficulty stopping drinking for that period, there could be more to your relationship with alcohol than meets the eye. Moderation Management is not an approach for someone who has been a dependent drinker in the past or who has significant withdrawal symptoms when they stop drinking. An example of this is what happened to the woman who first established Moderation Management. It turned out that she was a dependent drinker who several years later was convicted of vehicular manslaughter. An empty liquor bottle was found next to her following an auto accident in which two people died. She was not seriously injured. So do not drink if you feel you do not meet the definitions of a moderate drinker listed above.

(e)   *There is Another Option*

Ok, you can't or don't want to drink alcohol. What are your options? Another drug very similar to alcohol is Glucophage (*Greek for eats sugar*) or the generic metformin. This is a medication for patients with diabetes, but it is also being used to delay or prevent the onset of diabetes. It works by reducing insulin resistance through the reduction of the liver production of glucose. It appears to reduce heart attacks and cardiac death as well as cancer of the pancreas. See Chapter 18 Making Your Diabetes Go Away (in Volume II) for more details and the references.

Near the End of Volume I;

Congratulations!

Epilogue

Congratulations! You have made it this far. The reason this book seems to end so abruptly is because we are not yet finished. Knowing what to eat is only half of the solution. Volume II will explore much more about why we develop diseases and how to not only stay healthy but also heal our bodies and minds. This will include a discussion of how fear and guilt adversely affect our health (as shown by their strong association with heart disease, cancer and early death). You will develop understanding and learn techniques to help overcome adverse emotions and improve outcomes.

The Critical Information Presented in this Book:

Eating sugar and starch is death (but a little death is ok?)

Eating nuts is associated with increased longevity.

Ketosis appears to slow aging (which is a good thing).
> It also helps maintain and build lean body mass.
> Studies in animals and people show that our bodies are actually more efficient
> > and require less oxygen while exercising in ketosis.

Eating fatty fish and green leafy vegetables is hard to beat for a healthy meal.
> But avoid the farm-raised fish (not as good) and larger fish like tuna and swordfish
> > (mercury).
> If you can eat sardines you are probably tough enough to make it over 100 years old
> > (and still having sex).

Anger and depression kill (more about this in Volume II).
> So does excess alcohol consumption (but a little is actually good for you).

Limit your use of supplements; whole fresh food in a balanced diet is much better for you.
> But you just do not need the grains (unless you are crossing the damn desert!)

Milk makes more mucus in most of us
> (so if you have allergies avoid most dairy and citrus and sulfites in wine or wine
> > vinegar).

The best predictor of disease and death is the circumference of your waist.
> So don't check your weight, check your waist.
> If you avoid sugar and the starchy carbohydrates, you will lose weight.
> If you continue to avoid them, you will keep the weight off.

Fat is good for you. But try to make it olive oil, omega-3 fish oils, nut oils.

NUTRITIONAL CONTENT OF FOODS IN THE MEDITERRANEAN HUNTER-GATHERER DIET

Vegetables, Nuts and Fruit

Nuts and Seeds	**Cal**	**Fat**	**Mono**	**O3/O6** **Poly**	**Sat**	**Carb**	**Fiber**	**Protein**	**Chol**
Almonds, 30 nuts (1 oz)	180	16	11	0 / 4	1.5	7	4	7	0
Almond butter, 2 Tbs. (1 oz)	180	16	11	0 / 4	1.5	7	4	7	0
Brazil nuts, 8 medium (1 oz)	190	19	7	0 / 7	5	3	2	4	0
Cashews, 15 nuts (1 oz)	180	15	8	0 / 4	2.5	9	1	4	0
Cashew butter, 2 Tbs. (1 oz)	180	15	8	0 / 4	2.5	9	1	4	0
Flax seed, 3 Tbs. (1 oz)	140	10	2	6 / 2	1	11	8	5	0
Macadamia nuts, 16 nuts (1 oz)	220	20	11	0 / 4	5	3	2	3	0
Pecans, 14 halves (1 oz)	200	21	11	0 / 9	1	4	2	3	0
Pine nuts (1 oz)	190	18	5	0 / 11	2	6	2	8	0
Pistachios, 1 oz	180	16	3	0 / 11	2	8	2	6	0
Sunflower seeds, 1 oz	200	17	3	0 / 11	2	5	2	6	0
Walnuts, 14 halves (1 oz)	180	17	4	0 / 11	2	3	1.5	4	0
Mixed Nuts, 1 oz	180	16	8	0 / 6	2	7	3	5	0

Ground Nuts	**Cal**	**Fat**	**Mono**	**Poly**	**Sat**	**Carb**	**Fiber**	**Protein**	**Chol**
Peanuts, 35pcs (1 oz)	160	14	7	0 / 5	2	7	4	7	0
Peanut butter, 1Tbs. (1 oz)	160	14	7	0 / 5	2	7	4	7	0

Green Leafy Vegetables	**Cal**	**Fat**	**Mono**	**Poly**	**Sat**	**Carb**	**Fiber**	**Protein**	**Chol**
Arugula, 6 oz, 4 cups	50	0	0	0	0	8	4	6	0
Artichoke, 1 med.	60	0	0	0	0	8	6	6	0
Asparagus, 14 spears	60	0	0	0	0	12	6	6	0
Broccoli spears, 6 oz, 4 spears	50	0	0	0	0	8	4	6	0
Broccoli leaves, 6 oz, 1 cup	50	0	0	0	0	8	4	6	0
Brussel Sprouts, 6 oz, 12 med.	70	0	0	0	0	10	5	6	0
Cabbage (red), 3 oz, 1 cup	20	0	0	0	0	3	2	2	0
Cauliflower, 6 oz, 4 spears	50	0	0	0	0	8	4	6	0
Celery, 3 oz, 2 stalks	15	0	0	0	0	3	2	1	0
Collards, 3 oz, 1 cup	20	0	0	0	0	3	2	2	0
Dandelion greens, 1 cup	26	0	0	0	0	6	3	1	0
Endive, ½ whole	4	0	0	0	0	1		0	0
Kale, 3 oz, 1 cup	20	0	0	0	0	3	2	2	0
Leeks. 1/3 whole	20	0	0	0	0	3	2	2	0
Lettuce, red leaf , 4 cups, 6 oz	30	0	0	0	0	6	2	2	0
Scallions, 6 medium	15	1	0	0	0	3	1	0	Chol
Spinach, 6 oz, 4 cups	40	0	0	0	0	4	4	4	0
Turnip greens, 3 oz, 1 cup	30	0	0	0	0	3	2	2	0
Watercress, ½ cup	2	0	0	0	0	0	0	0	0

Vegetables, Nuts and Fruit

Fruit Vegetables	Cal	Fat	Mono	O3/O6 Poly	Sat	Carb	Fiber	Protein	Chol
Avocado, 1 medium	306	30	18	0/6	6	12	6	4	0
Cucumber, 1 medium	20	0	0	0	0	4	1	1	0
Eggplant, ¼ medium	11	0	0	0	0	3	1	0	0
Green beans, 1 cup	30	0	0	0	0	7	2	2	0
Olives, 6 olives	50	4	2	0 / 0	2	1	0	0	0
Okra, sliced 1 cup	36	0	0	0	0	8	3	3	0
Peas, ¾ cup	70	0	0	0	0	13	4	4	0
Peppers, sweet, 1 medium	18	0	0	0	0	4	1	1	0
Squash, summer, 1 cup	18	0	0	0	0	4	2	2	0
Tomato, 1 medium	20	0	0	0	0	8	2	2	0
Tomato, canned ½ cup	45	0	0	0	0	10	1	1	0
Water chestnuts, 4 oz can	25	0	0	0	0	5	1	1	0
Zucchini, 1 cup	18	0	0	0	0	4	2	2	0

Root Vegetables	Cal	Fat	Mono	Poly	Sat	Carb	Fiber	Protein	Chol
Carrot, 1 medium	30	0	0	0	0	5	2	1	0
Garlic, 1 clove pressed	4	0	0	0	0	1	1	0	0
Ginger, ¼ cup sliced	17	0	0	0	0	4	1	1	0
Onion, ½ cup chopped	32	0	0	0	0	7	2	1	0
Potato, 2"x5" baked	145	0	0	0	0	34	2	3	0
Sweet potato, 1 large	185	0	0	0	0	44	6	3	0

Miscellaneous Vegetables	Cal	Fat	Mono	Poly	Sat	Carb	Fiber	Protein	Chol
Mushrooms, 1 cup raw	24	0	0	0	0	4	1	2	0
Pepper rings, hot, 12 rings	5	0	0	0	0	1	0	0	0
Mustard- Stone ground, 1 Tsp.	14	1	0	0	0	1	0	1	0

Oils	Cal	Fat	Mono	O3/O6 Poly	Sat	Carb	Fiber	Protein	Chol
Canola oil, 1 Tbs.	130	14	8	2 / 3	1	0	0	0	0
Flax oil, 1 Tbs.	130	14	3	8 / 2	0	0	0	0	0
Olive oil, 1 Tbs.	130	14	10	0 / 2	2	0	0	0	0

Salad Dressings	Cal	Fat	Mono	O3/O6 Poly	Sat	Carb	Fiber	Protein	Chol
Olive oil/vinegar, 2 Tbs.	140	14	10	0 / 2	2	2	0	0	0
Flax oil/vinegar, 2 Tbs.	140	14	3	8 / 2	0	2	0	0	0
Canola oil mayonnaise, 1 Tbs.	100	11	6	0 / 3	1	0	0	0	5
"Real" mayonnaise, 1 Tbs .	100	11	3	0 / 7	1.5	0	0	0	5

Vegetables, Nuts and Fruit

Green Salads	Cal	Fat	Mono	Poly	Sat	Carb	Fiber	Protein	Chol
Green Salad, 6 oz, 4 cups	40	0	0	0	0	4	4	4	0
Olive Salad, 6 olives	50	4	2	0 / 0	2	1	0	0	0

Dips	Cal	Fat	Mono	Poly	Sat	Carb	Fiber	Protein	Chol
Almond butter, 1 Tbs.	180	16	11	0 / 4	1.5	7	4	7	0
Babaganoush, 2 Tbs.	50	3.5	1	0 / 2	0.5	5	1	2	0
Bean dip, 2 Tbs.	35	1	0	0	1	5	1	2	0
Cocktail sauce, ¼ cup	100	0	0	0	0	23	1	1	0
Guacamole, 2 Tbs.	30	3	2	0 / 1	0	2	0	0	0
Humus, 2 Tbs.	50	3.5	1	0 / 2	0.5	5	1	2	0

Fruits, fresh	Cal	Fat	Mono	Poly	Sat	Carb	Fiber	Protein	Chol
Apple, 1 small	81	0	0	0	0	21		0	0
Apricot, 3 medium	55	0	0	0	0	14	3	1	0
Banana, 1 medium, ripe	101	0	0	0	0	26	3	1	0
Blackberries, ½ cup	42	0	0	0	0	10	3	1	0
Blueberry, ½ cup	40	0	0	0	0	10	3	1	0
Cantaloupe, 1 cup cubed	48	0	0	0	0	12	0	1	0
Clementine/Tangerine, 1 medium	39	0	0	0	0	10	2	1	0
Grapefruit, ½ medium	43	0	0	0	0	11	1	1	0
Kiwi, 1 medium	46	0	0	0	0	11	3	1	0
Orange, 3" in diameter	90	0	0	0	0	20	3	2	0
Peach, 1 large	65	0	0	0	0	17	3	1	0
Pear, 1 medium	98	1	0	0	0	25	4	1	0
Pineapple, ½ cup fresh	41	0	0	0	0	11	0	1	0
Raspberries, ½ cup	35	0	0	0	0	9	4	1	0
Rhubarb, diced ½ cup	10	0	0	0	0	2	1	0	0
Strawberries, 1 cup halves	50	0	0	0	0	11	4	1	0

Fruits, dried	Cal	Fat	Mono	Poly	Sat	Carb	Fiber	Protein	Chol
Apricot, 3 medium	55	0	0	0	0	14	3	1	0
Figs, dried, 3 medium	90	0	0	0	0	23	3	1	0
Prunes, 3 medium	60	0	0	0	0	15	1	0	0
Raisins, ¼ cup packed	125	1	0	0	0	32	2	2	0

Fish, Poultry and Meats

Seafood	Cal	Fat	Mono	Poly	Sat	Carb	Fiber	Protein	Chol
Anchovies, 6 fillets	25	1.5	0	1 / 0	0	0	0	3	
Crabmeat (canned), 2 oz	45	1	0	1 / 0	0	0	0	8	50
Flounder, 6 oz	150	2	0	1 / 1	0	0	0	33	75
Haddock, 4 oz	99	1	0	1 / 0	0	0	0	21	65
Herring, kippered 3 oz	165	12	0	9 / 2	1	0	0	11	50
Mussels, 4 oz	98	3	0	2 / 1	0	4	0	14	32
Salmon, 4 oz	180	11	0	6 / 2	3	0	0	22	62
Salmon (smoked), 2 oz	130	9	0	5 / 1	2	0	0	11	30
Sardines, 3 oz, 1 can, olive oil	156	10	0	5 / 1	4	0	0	14	48
Scallops, 4 oz, ¾ cup	127	4	1	2 / 0	1	8	0	16	85
Shrimp, 4 oz	120	2	0	1 / 0	0	1	0	23	173
Tuna, 3 oz	105	2	0	2 / 0	0	0	0	22	37
Whitefish, 4 oz	153	7	0	3 / 2	1	0	0	22	68

Eggs	Cal	Fat	Mono	Poly	Sat	Carb	Fiber	Protein	Chol
Eggs, 2 large	140	9	3	1 / 2	3	1	0	12	426
Egg whites from 2 large eggs	60	0	0	0	0	2	0	12	0

Poultry	Cal	Fat	Mono	Poly	Sat	Carb	Fiber	Protein	Chol
Chicken breast									
-Skinless/boneless, 6 oz	190	4	0	0 / 2	2	0	0	37	120
-With skin and bone	270	18	4	0 / 4	10	1	0	32	120
Chicken thigh/leg/wing, 6 oz	375	30	8	0 / 4	18	0	0	25	150
Cornish game hen, 4 oz	270	18	4	0 / 4	2	0	0	30	170
Turkey breast, 6 oz	210	5	0	0 / 3	2	0	0	46	100
Turkey leg/thigh, 6 oz	310	17	4	0 / 3	10	0	0	44	138
Turkey bacon, ½ oz, 2 slices	42	2	0	0	1	0	0	6	20
Turkey sausage, Italian 4 oz	160	9	2	0 / 2	5	1	0	26	70

Beef/Pork/Lamb/Bison	Cal	Fat	Mono	Poly	Sat	Carb	Fiber	Protein	Chol
Bacon-Canadian, 3 slices	70	3	1	0	2	0	0	11	30
Bacon, 2 strips	60	5	2	0	3	0	0	4	10
Beef -Filet Mignon, 6 oz	278	20	11	0 / 1	8	0	0	48	130
Beef -Lean Ground, 6 oz	460	32	19	0 / 1	12	0	0	42	110
Beef -Roast, 6 oz	278	20	11	0 / 1	8	0	0	48	125
Beef -Sirloin, 6 oz	344	14	7	0 / 1	6	0	0	52	150
Beef –Tenderloin, 6 oz	278	20	11	0 / 1	8	0	0	48	135
Bison steak, 6 oz	210	4	0	1 / 1	2	0	0	48	120
Frankfurter, beef 1 link	142	13	6	0 / 1	6	1	0	5	27
Ham, cured w/out nitrites 6 oz	230	10	5	0 / 1	4	0	0	33	90
Lamb -Leg of, 6 oz	340	17	9	0 / 1	7	0	0	46	150
Lamb -Tenderloin, 6 oz	344	16	8	0 / 1	7	0	0	46	155
Pork -Tenderloin, 6 oz	392	18	9	0 / 1	8	0	0	54	135

Drinks and Snacks

Cocktail Hour	Cal	Fat	Mono	Poly	Sat	Carb	Fiber	Protein	Chol
Spirits 90 proof (1.5 oz)	105	0	0	0	0	0	0	0	0
Wine-dry 5 oz	85	0	0	0	0	3	0	0	0
Beer, Sam Adams equivalent 12 oz	146	0	0	0	0	13	1	1	0
Light beer									
-Sam Adams Light, 12 oz	99	0	0	0	0	10	1	1	0
-Miller High Life Light, 12 oz	99	0	0	0	0	7	0	1	0
-Coors and Amstel Light, 12 oz	99	0	0	0	0	5	0	1	0
-Miller Light, 12 oz	96	0	0	0	0	3	0	1	0
-Michelob Ultra, 12 oz	99	0	0	0	0	2	0	1	0

Beverages	Cal	Fat	Mono	Poly	Sat	Carb	Fiber	Protein	Chol
Cocoa, unsweetened, 1 Tbs.	20	1	0	0	1	3	1	1	0
Coffee, unsweetened brewed	4	0	0	0	0	1	0	0	0
Tea, unsweetened brewed	2	0	0	0	0	1	0	0	0
Colas and other sodas, 16 oz	201	0	0	0	0	51	0	0	0
Juices									
-Apple, 8 oz	116	0	0	0	0	29	0	0	0
-Cranberry, 2 oz unsweetened and diluted to 8 oz	54	0	0	0	0	14	0	0	0
-Grapefruit, 8 oz	94	0	0	0	0	22	0	0	0
-Orange, 8 oz	112	0	0	0	0	26	0	0	0
-V-8 Low Sodium, 8 oz	60	0	0	0	0	11	2	0	0
Soy milk- plain, 8 oz	130	4	1	0 / 1	1	13	0	10	0

Diet Breakfast Drinks	Cal	Fat	Mono	Poly	Sat	Carb	Fiber	Protein	Chol
Carnation Instant Breakfast, 1 can	210	3	0	0	0	34	1	12	10
Slim Fast, 1 can	220	2	0	0	0	48	5	7	10
Ensure Plus, 1 can	360	13	6	0 / 6	1	47	0	13	5

Candies and Snack Bars	Cal	Fat	Mono	Poly	Sat	Carb	Fiber	Protein	Chol
Chocolate, unsweetened, 1 oz	140	14	3	0 / 2	9	4	2	4	0
Chocolate, 70% unsweetened, 1 oz	136	10	2	0 / 2	6	12	2	3	0
Hershey's milk chocolate, 1.5 oz	200	12	3	0 / 2	7	21	1	3	10
Reese's peanut butter cup, 1.5 oz	250	14	4	0 / 2	8	25	1	5	5
Twix, 1 oz	140	7	3	0 / 1	4	19	0	1	0
Slim Fast Chewy Caramel	120	4	1	0 / 1	2	22	2	1	5
Granola bars	140	0	0	0	0	30	2	2	0
Power Bar, 1 bar	230	3	1	0 / 1	1	45	3	10	0
Pure Protein –Peanut butter, 1 bar	280	7	2	0 / 1	4	9	0	33	5

Sweeteners	Cal	Fat	Mono	Poly	Sat	Carb	Fiber	Protein	Chol
Stevia, 1 pack (sweet herb)	5	0	0	0	0	1	0	0	0
Sugar, 1 Tsp.	20	0	0	0	0	5	0	0	0
Molasses, blackstrap 1 Tbs.	42	0	0	0	0	11	0	0	0
Syrup, corn or Maple 1 Tbs.	61	0	0	0	0	16	0	0	0

Dairy

Dairy	Cal	Fat	Mono	Poly	Sat	Carb	Fiber	Protein	Chol
Butter, 1 Tbs.	102	12	4	0 / 0	8	0	0	0	31
Cheeses									
-Brie, 1 oz	94	8	3	0 / 0	5	0	0	6	28
-Cheddar, 1 oz	113	9	3	0 / 0	6	0	0	7	30
-Cream, 1 oz	98	10	4	0 / 0	6	1	0	2	30
-Goat, 1 oz	103	9	4	0 / 0	5	1	0	6	22
-Mozzarella, part skim 1 oz	79	6	2	0 / 0	4	1	0	5	15
-Muenster, 1 oz	103	8	3	0 / 0	5	0	0	7	27
-Swiss, 1 oz	105	8	3	0 / 0	5	0	0	8	25
Cottage cheese 1%, 1 oz	100	2	1	0 / 0	1	4	0	14	15
Creams									
-Heavy, 1 Tbs.	53	6	2	0 / 0	4	0	0	0	21
-Sour, 2 Tbs.	60	5	1	0 / 0	4	1	0	1	25
Milk, skim, 8 oz	80	0	0	0	0	12	0	8	3
Milk, whole, 8 oz	150	8	3	0 / 0	5	12	0	8	35
Yogurt (whole milk), 8 oz	150	8	2	0 / 0	5	11	0	9	31

Grain-Based Foods

Grain-Based Foods	Cal	Fat	Mono	Poly	Sat	Carb	Fiber	Protein	Chol
Bagel, 1 whole	190	1	0	1	0	41	12	6	0
Breads									
-12 Grain (Arnold), 2 slices	120	0	0	0	0	20	2	4	0
-Pita, ½ large	82	0	0	0	0	17	1	3	0
-Sourdough (Arnold), 2 slices	180	1	0	0	0	38	2	4	0
-Weightwatchers Multigrain, 2 sl.	82	2	0	0 / 1	0	14	4	4	0
-Wonderbread, 2 slices	110	1	0	0	0	20	1	30	
Crackers, wheat 6 pieces	140	6	0	0 / 5	1	19	1	2	0
Donut, glazed	170	10	0	0 / 8	2	19	0	2	0
Pancakes, 3 medium	200	3	1	0 / 1	1	40	2	6	15
Pasta noodles, 1 cup cooked	197	1	0	0	0	40	2	7	0
Pastry, Entenmann's Fat free, 1 bun	150	0	0	0	0	36	1	3	0

Grains and Beans	Cal	Fat	Mono	Poly	Sat	Carb	Fiber	Protein	Chol
Barley, ½ cup cooked	97	0	0	0	0	22	4	2	0
Beans,									
-Black, ½ cup cooked	114	0	0	0	0	20	7	8	0
-Chickpeas, ½ cup cooked	100	2	0	0	0	20	7	6	0
-Kidney, ½ cup cooked	112	0	0	0	0	20	7	8	0
-Lentil, ½ cup cooked	115	0	0	0	0	20	7	9	0
-Navy, ½ cup cooked	129	1	0	0	0	24	9	8	0
-Pinto, ½ cup cooked	116	0	0	0	0	22	8	7	0
Black-eyed peas, ½ cup cooked	90	0	0	0	0	19	5	7	0
Oats, rolled, ¼ cup	150	3	0	0 / 1	2	27	4	5	0
Rice, brown, ½ cooked	110	1	0	0/0	0	23	1	2	0
Rice cake, 1 plain	35	0	0	0	0	7	0	1	0
Soybeans, roasted, ¼ cup	202	11	0	0/9	2	29	2	15	0

Index